REHABILITATION OF THE
SEVERELY DISABLED

Compiled and Edited

by

William M. Jenkins
Robert M. Anderson
Wilson L. Dietrich

With a Foreword

by

Robert L. Saunders, Dean
College of Education
Memphis State University

Department of Special Education and Rehabilitation
College of Education
Memphis State University
Memphis, Tennessee

The conference which led to the publication of this book was supported by a grant from the Tennessee Division of Vocational Rehabilitation.

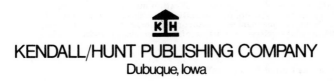

KENDALL/HUNT PUBLISHING COMPANY
Dubuque, Iowa

Contents

iii

Foreword

The publication of this book represents a major contribution to the field of vocational rehabilitation in the United States. The text has been adapted from the proceedings of a comprehensive conference on services for the severely disabled. The need for the conference was precipitated by passage of the Rehabilitation Act of 1973, which provided for increased services for severely disabled citizens. The contents of this book demonstrate that this was a fruitful conference. The College of Education is pleased that the development of the conference and the subsequent publication of this book was made possible by a grant from the Tennessee Division of Vocational Rehabilitation.

The content of the book was compiled and edited by Dr. William M. Jenkins, Dr. Robert M. Anderson, and Dr. Wilson L. Dietrich, Department of Special Education and Rehabilitation.

It is our hope that this compilation will assist rehabilitation counselors and others responsible for the various aspects of the rehabilitation of severely disabled citizens.

Robert L. Saunders, Dean
College of Education
Memphis State University

Preface

The Rehabilitation Act of 1973 requires that the state rehabilitation agencies serve the severely disabled. This greatly increases the responsibility of the total staff. The conference which led to the publication of this book was dedicated to the purpose of improving both our attitudes and our abilities to work with the severely disabled. We believe that the papers included in this compilation present an opportunity for practitioners to learn about new techniques and considerations relative to working with the severely disabled. I look forward to the successful implementation of the Rehabilitation Act and the impact it will have on services for seriously disabled people.

O. E. Reece
Assistant Commissioner
Division of Vocational Rehabilitation

Acknowledgments

In addition to the members of the Department of Special Education and Rehabilitation and the featured speakers, many persons contributed to the success of the conference and the publication of this book.

The cooperation and contributions of Dr. Billy M. Jones, President of Memphis State University, are deeply appreciated.

Very special thanks are due to Dr. Robert Saunders, Dean of the College of Education, Memphis State University, who provided the support and encouragement necessary for the success of the conference.

It is with gratitude that we acknowledge the interest and assistance of Dr. Benjamin E. Carmichael, Commissioner of Education, who delivered the Keynote Address and established a very positive style for the entire conference.

Appreciation is also extended to Mr. O. E. Reece, Mr. Jack Van Hooser, Mr. Frank E. Lee, Mr. James R. Brooks, and Mr. John Whitaker who provided leadership in the development of the conference and who served on the Conference Program Committee.

We are, indeed, indebted to Mr. Paul Hicks, who served on the Local Arrangement Committee, the many counselors and other professional personnel who participated in the conference, and the University's students who served as assistants and recorders during the panel session and in group discussions.

Our sincere appreciation is also given to Dorothy Lippmann, who undertook the difficult task of transcribing the conference tapes. Thanks are also due to Sara Odle, who helped to coordinate and manage the editing and preparation of the entire manuscript. In addition, Mrs. Odle wrote the abstracts which appear at the beginning of each paper.

Finally, we wish to thank the personnel of the Bureau of Educational Research and Services for editorial work and publication of the proceedings from which this book has been adapted.

William M. Jenkins
Robert M. Anderson
Wilson L. Dietrich

William M. Jenkins
Robert M. Anderson
and Wilson L. Dietrich

Overview and Perspectives

The Rehabilitation Act of 1973 was signed by President Nixon on September 26, 1973. The bill had previously been vetoed twice because of questions about fiscal responsibility and the extent to which programs should be expanded.[1] The basic goals or objectives of the Vocational Rehabilitation program were not at issue. Most of the controversy focused on the high level of authorization and the prospect that actual funding would not be forthcoming.

The major implication of the legislation for the conference described in this paper is that the new Act redirected the Vocational Rehabilitation program to focus on individuals with the "most severe handicaps" and required that each state plan show how persons receiving services would be selected to guarantee that those with the most severe handicaps would be served first.

Whitten pointed out that the new law does not establish any new program for the severely handicapped nor does it change the definition of the handicapped individual eligible for services in any significant way.[2] The new legislation does, however, require that each state agency must establish an order of priority for serving handicapped individuals and that severely disabled individuals will receive the *highest priority*.

According to Whitten the regulations developed pursuant to the Act represented a point of departure in the establishment of a definition of severe disability. A severely disabled individual was defined as "a handicapped individual who has a severe physical or mental disability which seriously limits his functional capacities (mobility, communication, self-care, or work skills) in terms of employability."

It is obvious that the Rehabilitation Act of 1973 represented a milestone in the vocational rehabilitation of severely disabled citizens in the United States. Emphasis on working with seriously handi-

1

capped persons and the training of personnel to work with such clients has consequently become of considerable concern to professional and nonprofessional personnel who work with the handicapped.

DEVELOPMENT OF THE CONFERENCE

For the past three years Memphis State University has continuously conducted programs that have been vital to rehabilitation counselors and other personnel in the Tennessee Division of Vocational Rehabilitation and the Mid-South region. The Division has been able to benefit from the experience of the MSU staff in various areas of training through short-term training courses and other training programs.

When the Division of Vocational Rehabilitation was confronted with the task of working with the more severely disabled citizens, the Assistant Commissioner of Vocational Rehabilitation, Mr. O.E. Reece, extended a proposal to the Department of Special Education and Rehabilitation at Memphis State University to develop a four-day workshop to focus on services for the severely disabled.

The staff at MSU agreed to plan, conduct, and evaluate a training program for the entire professional staff of the Division of Vocational Rehabilitation. At that time it was recognized that the DVR staff, comprised of approximately 375 professional people, would be required to commit more time and money to rehabilitation services for severely handicapped citizens than they had in years past.

The training program was subsequently conducted at the Holiday Inn Rivermont, Memphis, Tennessee, on August 27, 28, and 29, 1974. The staff of the Division of Vocational Rehabilitation represented the four regions of the State of Tennessee.

The general objectives of the inservice training program were:

1. To provide a high quality rehabilitation training program for the entire DVR professional staff.
2. To augment and enhance the general training program.
3. To intensify efforts during the forthcoming year in providing services to the more severely handicapped clients
4. To improve working relationships between the Department of Special Education and Rehabilitation, Memphis State University,

Memphis, Tennessee, and the Division of Vocational Rehabilitation.

PROGRAM DESCRIPTION

The objectives of the conference were achieved through a variety of lectures, panel discussions, and small group discussions. The general sessions included presentations on the interpretation of relevant sections of the Rehabilitation Act, information relative to certification, individualized programs, placement, on-the-job training, medical and psycho-social problems, and other content areas related to services for the severely disabled.

Only the central theme of each speaker, panel, or discussion group has been reported in this book, inasmuch as the total amount of material covered during the conference would have been too voluminous to be included in its entirety. Some material was not included because major portions of the tapes were distorted or inaudible. This occurred during sessions that included extensive audience participation.

For example, the panel discussion on the Rehabilitation Act of 1973 included questions and comments by various persons who spoke from a variety of scattered locations both on-stage and in the audience. Much of the tape on which this session was recorded could not be transcribed, and, therefore, the content is not included in these proceedings. Even though the material could not be included we would like to thank Mr. Jack Duncan, Mr. Joseph Owens, and Mr. Craig Mills for their significant contributions in leading the discussion about the Rehabilitation Act. Indeed, their reconstruction and analysis of the events which led to the presidential vetoes and subsequent passage of the Act constituted one of the highlights of the conference. In addition, they summarized and interpreted the major provisions of the Act and focused on practical implications for vocational rehabilitation. Mr. Duncan provided his interpretation from the perspective of his position as Chief Counsel for the Select Subcommittee on Education. Mr. Owens added input from his experience as Executive Director of the Council of State Administrators of Vocational Rehabilitation. Mr. Mills spoke from the dual vantage points of his position as State Director of DVR in Florida and as a participant in the oversight hearings during a very critical time in the history of the State-Federal Rehabilitation Program.

At the completion of the conference an evaluation form was completed by each participant. The responses were tabulated and are included in the last section of this report, "Conclusions and Implications."

Notes

1. M. L. LaVor and J. C. Duncan, "Rehabilitation Act of 1973, P.L. 93-112," *Exceptional Children*, XL (1974), 443-49.

2. E. B. Whitten, "The Rehabilitation Act of 1973," *Journal of Rehabilitation*, XL (1974)2, 39-40.

Benjamin E. Carmichael

Keynote Address

Current state and federal legislation emphasizes the rights of all individuals to appropriate services appropriately provided. Comprehensive planning for the delivery of such services to the handicapped must include provision for the development of personal and emotional characteristics, for integration as a contributing member of the community, and for job competency. The interface between the Division of Vocational Rehabilitation, Vocational Education, Research and Development, and other agencies of the State Department of Education results in more effective planning of and provision for such comprehensive services for the handicapped in the state of Tennessee.

During the past two weeks I have had the opportunity to participate with several school systems in their inservice education programs prior to the beginning of school. I am enjoying these activities perhaps more than any activities of this sort that I have ever participated in because I think I have the opportunity this year to really implement the work of the State Department of Education and the work of our several school systems across this state. I hope to be engaged in sharing some of the most meaningful activities and work experiences that I have ever known in education in Tennessee. And these activities, I think, are very closely related to the kinds of objectives that you have and the kind of work, in many instances, that you are doing in Tennessee. I have tried to project our responsibilities in terms of the joint effort that we must make with the several local agencies and school systems across this state if we are indeed going to be able to deliver the kinds of services that are required by the very special groups that we serve. I have tried to mobilize the State Department of Education and all of its units and division in terms of the very sincere interests that we have in these activities. We want to be characterized as persons who are not interested in regulatory functions only, or even to any large extent. We have the same interest in service and people that other agency and school

5

systems have, and we are willing to roll up our sleeves and engage in the tough work of serving.

The department is now composed of about 3,900 people. We have in this department three technical institutes, which represent the closest that the department now comes, under the State Board of Education, to anything in higher education, and that relationship is only in terms of some instruction that can be transferred to colleges and universities. There are twenty-six area vocational schools and more than 160 vocational centers and units being projected across the state as part of a comprehensive vocational education program designed to serve at least 50 per cent of all high school youngsters and to provide service at the post-secondary level to those who need it. There is the Division of Vocational Rehabilitation, of course, and also the divisions of Vocational Education and of Library and Archives, and those divisions combined into a major bureau of special services with about six or seven other units that necessarily function under the State Department of Education and the State Board of Education. There are three major divisions that relate directly to the operation of the 146 school systems across the state. The function of the Division of School System Management and Planning is to work almost on a daily basis with the school superintendents and boards of education to help plan and manage the school systems of the State.

The Division of Research and Development has become larger than any educational research and development center or laboratory across this country. I am extremely proud of this division because I happen to believe that change can be effected only through a very sound program of research and development, a type of work perhaps requiring more capability and professional development and training than any other part of education. If I am correct in my belief that great change is needed in education, then we must see a genuine effort, based on good research, to develop new practices and procedures through tedious and careful development of products that can deliver the services required in education across this state. I am going to talk about some of the very important kinds of things that are included in the R and D mold at this time, and particularly those that I think are most significant to you. I do this because I think everything that I am going to talk about speaks to the basic theme of this conference, that of "individual rights," the rights of individuals who, up to this time, for the most part, have been relegated to secondary citizenship status.

In many instances large numbers of people have not been able to get into the mainstream of life because it seems that we've been concerned with those who are much easier to serve and those who probably can best get our attention. As I think of the amendments to the 1973 Vocational Rehabilitation Act, it seems to me that they are saying to us from the federal level the same things we have heard at the state level—that everyone has equal rights to education and rehabilitation. I think that there is no question regarding the emphasis that we, as educators, have placed on career education. I've studied this trend considerably. I don't happen to be one who "jumps on the bandwagon" because somebody comes along with a new phrase. I think that the concept of career education deserves careful analysis if we are going to fulfill the excellent intentions implicit in the concept.

As I sat in conference with Secretary Marland, former Secretary Works, and other persons trying to define career education, I found myself "turning them off" and attempting to write my own definition. I did this because I think we all need to try to state what we think, what we feel, what we believe, or what something means to us. I reduced the definition to this kind of thing which I think includes and involves you so much. A career, or career education, is the preparation of a life to live. A life to live consists, it seems to me, of three major kinds of things; that is, as we prepare someone for that life, we have three all-important kinds of things to be concerned about. One of those is always the development of those personal characteristics which contribute to society as a person works, which contribute to the building of the individual as he lives, which help him to be content, to be acceptable, which help him get the kinds of recognition and build the kind of confidence that he needs. This has to be one of the very vital kinds of preparation that we give.

Second, I think we have to think of every individual as needing preparation to live in communities, to live among us, for us to live with as neighbors. I don't know of anything of much significance that can really be accomplished individually or apart from the community or the group in which we live and work. It's obvious to me that the development of civic awareness, social responsibility, the ability to be a part of the total society, stressing the importance of pulling together and of making decisions together has to be the second, all-important kind of preparation for a career.

And then last, of course, there has to be the preparation for work. Whether it's professional or nonprofessional, I think it is not over-generalizing at all to say that all of us must prepare to do something worthwhile. In my lifetime I've known a few fortunate or unfortunate individuals, whichever way you might want to clasify them, who did not appear to have to work. But I have never found those ind-viduals over a long period of time being very successful or being able to maintain or further develop the other two very important kinds of characteristics and capabilities. So, I don't think it's over-generalizing at all to say that all of us need preparation for work.

To pursue this line of thinking just a little further, however, we hear a lot of verbalization about what career education means. We generally define career education as meaning all of education, and we say we don't want to confuse it with just one little **part of educa-tion** (we're referring usually to vocational education); and we don't, that's true. I don't want to imply that I would think otherwise, but I do want us to think just a little more basically about the true meaning of this. Hopefully we want to establish career education in our communities as a total part of the education and rehabilitation of people. Has our education ever been directed toward anything other than those three kinds of things? I've been in education several years now. I've had some very deep associations, and, as I have known people who are in the various social fields, I am convinced that we've always tried to prepare a person in those kinds of things which I've just mentioned. We've failed, perhaps, in many instances, or certainly done less than we wished to do. What has been our great deficiency? Again, risking over-simplification, I think we have not actually prepared people vocationally to do the kinds of jobs that are available. It's been easier to do the other. It's been less expensive to do the other, and consequently it has been very easy for us to project our work and our efforts to keep ourselves pretty well concerned only with the kinds of education that seemed to serve those who were pursuing careers. I think it's only now that we really, in a very sincere way, are drawing ourselves back to the careful consideration of our responsibilities to all persons.

These kinds of things in education—from kindergarten to compensatory education oriented in the home, the education of the handicapped, as provided for in Chapter 839 of the Comprehensive Vocational Education Act, the community programs for indigent and neglected children, now a state-wide leading program covering the first three grades, the emphasis upon services to the deaf here in the West Tennessee area—all of these seem to be supporting and trying to guarantee the rights of individuals to the same opportunities of reaching and succeeding in their careers as others have. I've had some very interesting experiences with regard to 839, just as you will have interesting experiences in serving the severely handicapped or in rehabilitation. The first comments on this act, especially those about a year ago, were always, "Well, you know, we have no business projecting ourselves into this kind of comprehensive service for handicapped people when we are not yet serving normal people adequately." I was always responding, "I'm sorry, but that isn't the question." The individual rights of people are not to be denied until the rights of some other people are supposedly completely met. It is not a matter of being eligible after we have accomplished or achieved this kind of thing for others. It is a matter of being eligible—based upon the fact that they are individuals who have the same rights to our services as any other individuals for just that purpose.

As we in the field of education strive toward programs that start at a very early age, as we think in terms of those identifications, as we think of participating in that total effort, I hope that we can begin seeing, down the road somewhere in the not-too-distant future, the opportunity to have very comprehensive, very well planned systems of services for all such people. We need your help tremendously, speaking of "we" from the standpoint of education—and I really apologize for doing that because it's not a "we and they" or "we and you" kind of thing we are talking about. If we view this as a spectrum beginning with trying to reach into the homes of handicapped children by the ages of one and two, getting proper identification, starting the kind of training that is needed, then perhaps we can deal adequately with some of the problems that are almost impossible to deal with when they reach the level of responsibility where you put forth effort.

We've been fortunate in having the assistance that you in rehabilitation have given to education in the past few years. The beginning of pilot programs at high school levels was mentioned earlier.

You are now serving children in high schools in some thirty-four systems across the state, in 166 schools as I recall. You have about 5,000 youngsters involved, and last year you produced or graduated from these programs some 750 youngsters who went into profitable employment. You moved in with a real service. The total task is not yours, but I am extremely happy you are a part of it, because I have seen so many instances where, in my opinion, you delivered better than we were able to deliver. You deliver better because you have some better perceptions of how to really develop people along these areas. You're very down to earth with the kinds of things you do.

Now, as we are trying to put together a total comprehensive program across the state involving not only the Department of Education, but also other departments providing related services to handicapped people, we find ourselves in the department doing the best work that has ever been done. In looking at the part of this total task that Vocational Rehabilitation can assist us with and the part of it that Vocational Education can assist us with, we find a particular relationship between your work and that of Vocational Education. Through this relationship we are about to establish the capability of accelerating the work that you will do. In the proposed center you are already working together. I see great things coming from that. I think you will get your basic experience there. While that is rather well institutionalized, I would expect to see you, in the not-too-distant future, spreading out across the state and finding ways of reaching the same kind of objectives in less than fully institutionalized settings.

As you proceed in this conference, I hope there will be things of this sort, in addition to the specific study that you are here for, that you will think about and you'll devote attention to.

No doubt you're going to have an excellent conference. As many of you perhaps know, we use in the Department of Education a weekly report from every division or unit in the department. That report, briefly, tells us the significant things that occurred during the past week, and it reports the major kinds of things that are going to happen in the coming week. I was very interested in the one coming from Vocational Rehabilitation last Friday. It reported that one of the finest staff conferences the division has experienced in its fifty-three years of operation will be held this week, and I believe this.

Craig Mills

The Development of the Rehabilitation
Acts of 1973 and 1974

This original paper was solicited specifically from the author for inclusion in this book. In the article, significant issues, developments, and events leading to presidential vetoes and subsequent passage of the Act and the Amendments of the following year are discussed and analyzed. Major provisions of the Act are summarized.

With the Rehabilitation Act of 1973 and the Rehabilitation Amendments of 1974 an accomplished fact, it is difficult to go back and put together all the unusual circumstances that took place over a period of nearly four years in the development and final approval of this rehabilitation legislation. But these were significant events that shaped the course of rehabilitation in America and will continue to affect the future of rehabilitation programs for handicapped people for many years to come. Serious issues between the legislative and executive branches of the government were brought to the forefront. Relationships between state and the federal government became a real issue. And the role of handicapped people themselves in determining their destiny in this country became more clearly defined as a result of the several years of struggle and debate over the rehabilitation legislation. For all these reasons it is therefore important for anyone who would try to understand where rehabilitation is today to also understand the complicated forces that influenced the development of this legislation.

Perhaps the first important event to consider was the need for renewal of the Rehabilitation Act in 1970. The statutory authorizations in the Act usually provided coverage for a specific period of time and gave the legal basis for the appropriation of funds during that period of coverage. In the final year of the authorization in the Act, the administration through the Department of Health, Education and Welfare would submit legislation to provide new authorizations and would use these occasions to propose amendments to the Act in keeping with the needs of a dynamic and developing program.

For reasons known only to the Administration, the Rehabilitation Act was allowed to expire with no recommendations being sent to the Congress. Although the rehabilitation organizations which had traditionally worked closely with the Rehabilitation Services Administration urged the submission of new legislation, this was not forth-coming. To avoid a serious gap in statutory support for the program, the Committee on Education and Labor of the House of Representatives submitted legislation to extend the Act for an additional year and to allow time in 1971 for legislation to be developed and introduced.

Again the Administration failed to submit legislation although the National Rehabilitation Association, the Council of State Administrators of Vocational Rehabilitation, and other rehabilitation-related organizations had worked closely with the Rehabilitation Services Administration and the Social and Rehabilitation Service in the Department of Health, Education and Welfare to outline constructive changes in the Act which appeared to be necessary and timely.

It is difficult now to present any satisfactory hypothesis to explain the lack of action on the part of the Administration. A variety of explanations have been given by knowledgeable observers of the scene. These may be worth considering in order to get some understanding of the political climate that existed at that time.

First, the Social and Rehabilitation Service had been created administratively in 1967 by the Secretary of HEW, John Gardner, to try to bring about a rehabilitation emphasis in the welfare and social service programs of the Department. Miss Mary Switzer, the highly successful Commissioner of the Office of Vocation Rehabilitation, was made the Administrator of the Social and Rehabilitation Service. The Rehabilitation Services Administration was made a part of this huge federal agency. But in the next few years, Secretary Gardner resigned and Miss Switzer retired in 1970. People with a different program philosophy and different priorities replaced them. Many people in the field of rehabilitation felt that there was no longer a rehabilitative emphasis in the Welfare and Social programs of HEW, but that there was a dramatic change to give a social direction to rehabilitation. Eligibility for rehabilitation services was opened to the disadvantaged, to the socially handicapped, and to public offenders through a change in regulations. As a consequence, the special resources of the Rehabilitation Act which provided for research and demonstration grants, innovation and expansion grants, special projects, and training, were controlled by the Social and Rehabilitation Service and were used to further the program emphasis for socially disadvantaged people. The emphasis was shifted from physically handicapped and mentally handicapped, and the major interest of the Department seemed to wing away from rehabilitation programs. This shift was given as one possible explanation for the lack of effort in rehabilitation legislation.

A related explanation was that the Rehabilitation Services Administration had made legislative proposals which it could not get cleared through SRS or the office of the Secretary of HEW. Here again, the possible explanation was that SRS and HEW were more concerned with welfare reform legislation which consumed their time and interests while rehabilitation legislation was given a low interest and a low priority.

In the light of subsequent events revealed at the Congressional oversight hearings on the rehabilitation program in 1973, many people in rehabilitation felt that the lack of action on the part of the administration represented a planned and concerted effort on the part of HEW to downgrade or abolish the vocational rehabilitation program for the handicapped in favor of a cash benefits, expanded welfare system.

Whatever the combination of these factors or circumstances, the leadership for the introduction of rehabilitation legislation had to come from outside the administration.

The individuals and groups who had offered assistance to the administration worked together with the National Rehabilitation association and the staff of the House Committee on Education and Labor to develop legislation. This bill, H.R. 8395, was introduced on May 13, 1971, by Congressman Carl D. Perkins of Kentucky, the Chairman of the full committee, and twenty-three other members representing broad bi-partisan support.

This legislation together with other related bills to amend the Vocational Rehabilitation Act became the vehicle for extensive hearings in the House. These hearings were conducted by Congressman John Brademas of Indiana, the Chairman of the Select Subcommittee on Education of the Committee on Education and Labor of the House of Representatives. These hearings were conducted in January and February of 1972 and a bill was promptly passed by the House. In its committee report on these hearings the House Committee issued a clarion call to the Rehabilitation Service Administration to abandon its emphasis on serving the socially handicapped and disadvantaged population and to give first priority to the physically and mentally handicapped.

The Senate Subcommittee on the Handicapped of the Committee on Labor and Public Welfare conducted extensive hearings on May 15th, 18th, 22nd and June 2nd and 6th, 1972. These hearings were open to all the major public and voluntary agencies and organizations for the handicapped. Lengthy oral and written testimony was presented covering every phase of rehabilitation service for handicapped people. This included lengthy documentation on the needs of severely disabled people with handicaps of blindness, deafness, cerebral palsy, mental retardation, mental illness, spinal cord injuries and other severe disabilities. It also included testimony and documentation on the needs for rehabilitation facilities, the need for training programs for skilled rehabilitation manpower, and the need for research and demonstration grant programs. Consternation was expressed by witnesses who indicated that rehabilitation resources in training and research were being diminished and that severely handicapped people were not able to get the services they needed. From the Senate came additions to the bill which would have provided for an entirely new but limited authority to provide rehabilitation services to the most severely handicapped persons without vocational potential but who might benefit substantially from comprehensive rehabilitation services.

Out of this crucible of Congressional study and broad public testimony including testimony from handicapped people and organizations for the handicapped, the House and Senate conferees presented rehabilitation legislation which received unanimous support from both houses of Congress in October, 1972.

It was therefore rather shocking to the rehabilitation movement to find that this legislation born of so much Congressional consideration and public support was unacceptable to the Administration and was given a "pocket veto" when President Nixon refused to sign the bill as the Congress adjourned for the general elections.

The explanation given for the veto included the proposed expansion of the Rehabilitation Act to include the limited title authorizing rehabilitation services to the most severely handicapped individuals without vocational potential.

This provision was considered in the veto message to open the door to making the rehabilitation program a program of medical services for the chronically ill. This and other provisions in the law were criticized as being inflationary, and the veto prior to the elections of the fall of 1972 was used as a vehicle to promote the theme of fiscal responsibility and control of inflation by the administration. When the Congress reconvened in January, 1973, there was insufficient support to override a presidential veto.

A variety of compromise bills was offered and there was extensive administration effort to delete major portions of the legislation which would have added any new service programs to the Act, and efforts were made to reduce substantially the fiscal authorizations.

After substantial changes were made in the law and major concessions were made by supporters of the legislation, a new bill, H.R.-17, was cleared by bi-partisan conferees of both houses and received almost unanimous support by both houses in March, 1973. This legislation followed the presidential election of 1972 and the sweeping changes in the administration following the landslide election of President Nixon.

This first Rehabilitation Act of 1973 was again vetoed by the President, and the Congress was not able to override the veto. This action in early 1973 left the rehabilitation program without extension of the Act and without authorizations. The prospects for any early passage of legislation acceptable to the Administration appeared bleak.

A new administrative team in the Social and Rehabilitation Service proceeded from a position of strength to advocate substantial cut-backs in support programs of research and demonstration, expansion and innovation grants, rehabilitation facilities and training, and proposed decreases in basic grants to states for rehabilitation services.

Throughout 1973 the negotiations went forward slowly, and finally in August of 1973 a Compromise Rehabilitation Act cleared a Conference Committee and was passed by both houses of the Congress. Although the administration had substantial reservations on some of the Administration requirements of the Act, the reduction of fiscal authorizations appeared to meet the Administration's requirements and Public Law 89-312, the Rehabilitation Act of 1973, was approved on September 26, 1973.

To understand some of the provisions in the Rehabilitation Act of 1973 it would be necessary to explain that on August 3, 1973, Oversight Hearings were conducted before the Select Subcommittee on Education and Labor of the House of Representatives on Future Directions of the Rehabilitation Services Administration. In these hearings officials of HEW, SRS and RSA were called upon to explain certain planning documents which were alleged to have called for the replacement of the state-federal vocational rehabilitation program by a cash benefits program which would provide resources to the handicapped individual rather than provide comprehensive services.

Administration officials were also questioned extensively on an administration proposal to discontinue support for specialized training of rehabilitation manpower.

These oversight hearings were followed by additional oversight hearings by the Select Subcommittee on Education and Labor on November 30, 1973, when representatives of the Council of State Administrations of Vocation Rehabilitation and representatives of the Council of Rehabilitation Counselor Educators were called to testify with representatives of HEW, SRS and RSA. This second oversight hearing focused on Congressional dissatisfaction with the way the Social and Rehabilitation Service was administering the Vocational Rehabilitation Act and the Rehabilitation Service Administration.

The testimony of the Council of State Administration of Vocational Rehabilitation revealed a lack of SRS support for Research and Demonstration, Innovation and Expansion Grant Programs and Training. Concern was expressed about the use of resources under the Rehabilitation Act to further the priorities of SRS to the neglect of the needs of handicapped people. Special concerns were expressed on the way SRS had promoted organizational arrangements in the states which appeared to be in violation of the Federal Rehabilitation Act and which diminished the effectiveness of specific programs for handicapped people. CSAVR representatives called for strict compliance with the rehabilitation act by SRS officials to insure that handicapped people received the specialized services they needed, and that resources under the act were used for the benefit of handicapped people.

Representatives of the Council of Rehabilitation Counselor Educators presented testimony in favor of the preservation of specialized rehabilitation counselor education programs under the law which SRS had proposed to phase out.

The Select Subcommittee called upon HEW and SRS officials to explain and justify the approval of a state plan in a state which appeared to be out of compliance with substantial requirements of the Rehabilitation Act. The response given by the SRS officials that approval of the state plan was in keeping with Administration policy rather than compliance with the law probably served as a basis for Congressional determination to mandate organization changes in HEW and to direct the removal of the Rehabilitation Services Administration from the Social and Rehabilitation Service. This established the basis for the Rehabilitation Act of 1974.

Before discussing the events connected with the passage of the Rehabilitation Act of 1974, it might be helpful to give some brief discussion of the major new provisions of the Rehabilitation Act of 1973.

First, it established the Rehabilitation Service Administration in HEW and mandated that it be headed by a Commissioner appointed by the President. It further prohibited any delegation of the authority of the Commission to anyone not responsible directly to the Commission unless the Secretary of HEW first submitted a plan for approval by the Congress. It mandated that funds appropriated under the Act should be used only for the programs, personnel and administration of programs carried out under the Act.

This provision is highlighted here because the failure of SRS to heed this statutory admonition from the Congress resulted in a key provision of the Rehabilitation Act of 1974.

The new act gave priority to service to institutions with severe handicapped while retaining the eligibility requirement of a vocational goal for each person served.

Participation by the handicapped person or his representative in the development of his rehabilitation program was assured by the requirement of an individualized written rehabilitation program for each rehabilitation client.

It authorized advanced funding to afford adequate planning for a subsequent year.

Congress expressed its continuing concern for the most severely handicapped who do not have vocational potential by authorizing a special study of this population.

It also authorized an extensive study of rehabilitation workshops.

The Congress reaffirmed its support for research and training by retaining the statutory and fiscal authority for these support programs.

New provisions included authority to provide mortgage insurance for the construction of rehabilitation facilities, establishment of client assistance pilot projects, and the authority to conduct studies on neglected areas.

A major new Title V called for an intergovernmental committee on employment of handicapped individuals by governmental agencies; the creation of an architectural barriers and transportation barriers compliance board, the requirement of affirmative action plans in the employment of handicapped persons by organizations using federal contracts of $2500 or more; and a provision for non-discrimination against otherwise qualified handicapped persons in work conducted under federal contracts.

In summary this new law gave a new thrust to priority service for individuals with severe mental and physical handicaps and directed emphasis away from the SRS priorities of serving the disadvantaged and socially handicapped.

The law gave considerable new emphasis to the recognition of the needs and rights of handicapped individuals and established safeguards to insure their participation in decisions affecting their destiny.

In the months immediately following the passage of the Rehabilitation Act of 1973 it did not appear to the Congress that the administration was giving serious consideration to the administration requirements that the Rehabilitation Service Administration be administered by a Commissioner who was fully responsible for the program. This concern was magnified as a result of the oversight hearings in November and December of 1973.

There was an obvious need to make some clarifications in the Rehabilitation Act of 1973, and there was a strong support developing for the passage of the Randolph-Sheppard Act Amendments on the vending stand program for the blind in federal buildings and installations. There was also substantial support in the Congress for the creation of an office for Handicapped Individuals in HEW, and the authorization of a White House Conference on the Handicapped. This combination of factors brought about amendments to the Rehabilitation Act of 1973, which were passed by both houses of the Congress late in 1974.

Again the Rehabilitation Act was subjected to a presidential veto on the basis that the requirement to remove the Rehabilitation Services Administration from SRS constituted an invasion of prerogatives of the Administrative branch of government. Once again the presidential veto was a "pocket veto" during a period of congressional recess.

This time an aroused Congress and overwhelming support by every segment of the rehabilitation movement resulted in an override of the veto by an almost unanimous vote. This strong expression of concern for handicapped people and for the preservation of the state-federal rehabilitation program as a specialized service for handicapped people probably represents the coming of age of this distinctive service program.

Because legal questions were raised about the action to override a "pocket veto," the Congress took immediate action to reintroduce the legislation and pass it anew on December 7, 1974. In the face of this resounding support for the Act the President allowed it to become law.

This law, the Rehabilitation Amendments of 1974, PL 93-516, mandated the removal of the Rehabilitation Services Administration from the Social and Rehabilitation Service within sixty days. It also included the Randolph-Sheppard Act amendments for the blind.

The administration moved promptly to transfer the Rehabilitation Services Administration to the Office of Human Development headed by a Deputy Secretary of HEW, and to give authority for the administration of the provisions of the Act to the Commissioner of the Rehabilitation Services Administration.

This change at the central office level in Washington was also accompanied by a corresponding change in the ten HEW Regional Offices throughout the country where RSA Regional Rehabilitation

Directors responsible to the Commissioner of the Rehabilitation Services Administration have been located in the Regional Office of Human Development, HEW.

All administration ties with the Social and Rehabilitation Service have been terminated. Organizationally, RSA appears to be in a position in 1975 to carry out the Congressional mandates for the program.

This process of developments of legislation covered a period of nearly four years. While it was a long and agonizing process there were some secondary benefits which may have long run value for the program.

The extensive hearings before both houses of the Congress afforded an opportunity for nearly every segment of the rehabilitation movement to participate in the development of the legislation. The voice of consumers and organizations of the handicapped were heard. The Congress was impressed by this testimony and reflected this in the committee reports and in the legislation.

The series of vetoes and rehandling of the Rehabilitation Act by the Congress resulted in more members of the Congress becoming acquainted with the details of the program. The widespread public support for the legislation resulted in the greatest grass-roots involvement in support of rehabilitation programs and facilities in the history of the movement. As a result, there was a substantial increase in public awareness of the program and of the needs of handicapped people. This public exposure may have opened a new era of concern for the rights and needs of physically handicapped and mentally handicapped people with severe vocational handicaps.

William M. Jenkins

Counselor Certification

Planning toward certification of rehabilitation counselors has been going forward for a number of years. Endorsement of such certification has been given by national rehabilitation organizations and committees. Standards and criteria have been developed by the National Commission on Rehabilitation Counselor Certification. Lack of adequate communication to counselors of the goals, procedures, and criteria for participation in the certification process has caused much confusion.

An explanation is given of reasons for the grandfathering year and the counselor's role in evaluating and developing the final form of the certifying test. Eligibility requirements, application deadlines, and locations of testing centers are given. A breakdown of the expenses involved in test construction and certification procedure shows the use made of the application and testing fees.

In developing the program of the conference, it was our concern to present some topics that would be relevant and timely, and of course the legislation that was discussed this morning, the 1973 Rehabilitation Act, was at the top of our list. There are some other topics that I think are also relevant. I decided to discuss counselor certification after I received a Vocational Rehabilitation Newsletter that indicated that I was supposed to be the expert on counselor certification in Tennessee. I didn't know that until I read it, and I think John Whitaker is the one who put it in there. So I decided that if I was to be the source of information, then perhaps I had better learn something about it. Now, I know that this is a very controversial topic—counselor certification. I hope that none of you throw tomatoes at me, or eggs, or cabbage, or whatever. I want you to know that I am taking a neutral stand on counselor certification, at least for the purpose of this talk. We also thought that perhaps we should discuss counselor certification because we've been getting a lot of letters from angry counselors—counselors who appear to be confused, counselors who feel that they have been given incorrect information. So the whole purpose of this presentation is to try to clear up some of that confusion, if possible.

I heard the other day that when encountering a problem you might deal with this problem in one of four ways. I think that we as rehabilitation counselors or rehabilitation workers perhaps utilize all of these approaches. One is protocol, and I imagine that this is the method used by our distinguished guest from Washington. If that doesn't work, then alcohol, and I think probably that this is the answer that a lot of rehab people seek. I know I find solace in it occasionally, and a lot of you did last night. If that doesn't work, then Hadacol, and then damn-it-all. And a lot of counselors have said "damn-it-all" to counselor certification. I'm hoping that perhaps I can give you some information today that will enable you to evaluate it a little more objectively. It seems that the committee or the Commission on Counselor Certification is constantly changing policy. One week they do one thing, another week they've done something else, and this is what a lot of counselors have been a little concerned about. I called the Commission this morning and asked if they had made any additional policy changes. I'm serious when I say this, because I did actually call them, and they indicated that there had been no changes since yesterday afternoon at 5 o'clock, so I think I have the most up-to-date information available.

Now in order to discuss counselor certification, it probably would be helpful to give you just a little background information. As you probably know, counselor certification has been in the planning stage for a number of years, but the major effort toward the development of the actual procedure began in the spring of 1970 when the American Rehabilitation Counseling Association (ARCA) and the National Rehabilitation Counselor Association (NRCA) together appointed a Joint Certification Committee. The committee was chaired by G. D. Karns who at that time was Coordinator of Rehabilitation Counselor Education at the University of Texas. Out of the joint committee development came the now often quoted Karns report. As a result of this committee effort, additional involvements have occurred that have pushed counselor certification pretty close to the middle of the national rehabilitation stage. One of these developments has been the endorsement of counselor certification by the National Rehabilitation Association, the parent organization; another has been the formation of the National Commission on Rehabilitation Counselor Certification. Out of this commission have come standards and criteria for Rehabilitation Counselor Certification. The standards and criteria are what I would like to discuss for the next few minutes.

The purpose of this discussion is not to sell you on counselor certification. I don't think that certification requires a sales pitch from me. It either stands or falls on its own merit as perceived by each individual counselor and on its relevancy to the counselor. I would like to try and clear up some confusion that seems to exist, and believe me there does exist a lot of confusion about this procedure, not only in Tennessee, but also across the entire country. I think that even the Commission on Certification will admit to some poor journalism in the beginning and a failure, during the first year, to communicate adequately to the membership the goals, procedures, and criteria for participation in the certification process. For this reason many counselors have literally become unbridled, angry, and disenchanted over the issue and in many respects turned off by the whole thing. I suppose some of the confusion can be accounted for by the mere fact that any new endeavor, particularly one as controversial as counselor certification, would have some ambiguous or controversial parts in the beginning. Some of this confusion is likely to continue during this grandfathering year. I think this is another reason that it is critical for us to discuss counselor certification now, because we are into the grandfathering year which will expire July 1, 1975.

I would like to make one point here. We do have a diverse group—we have counselors, we have training center managers, we have administrators and supervisors, we have some university people, we have some disability examiners, and we have others, and I would like for this presentation to be directed to all of you. Hopefully you will consider it relevant. Any trial run or field test of a new procedure is likely to produce some inconsistencies, because the primary objective of a field test, and that is what the grandfathering year is designed for, is to develop standard operating procedures (SOP), and those of you who have been in the service know what this means. These procedures will ultimately eliminate problems and confusion and hopefully refine the whole process. As you probably know, the first examination was given July 19th of this year, and some of you participated at that time.

In developing any new instrument that is to be used for assessment purposes, it is imperative that the instrument have relevance and validity and, as this applies to us, relevance and validity regarding the practice of rehabilitation counseling. Now who should have input into the development of this validity? The Commission on Certification says "You" should have this input, and this is why you are being required to take an examination. They don't call it an examination any more; it's a very poor term and scares a lot of people. They're now calling it a field review. This is the reason why you are being asked to participate during this grandfather year by taking the examination. Because, after all, it is you the counselor, or some colleague of yours, or some future counselor, whose competency will be tested, and it is you who will help develop this procedure to be administered after July of 1975. Each person being grandfathered will be asked to evaluate the appropriateness of each item as to content, relevance, and validity regarding what he perceives to be the knowledge required of a rehabilitation counselor. In effect, you are doing this during the grandfathering year to evaluate the test rather than having the test evaluate you. Now doesn't that sound good? How many of us like to be tested? There will be no cutoff scores. You cannot fail this examination. Your scores will not be compared to some criterion referenced group for the purpose of determining success or failure. The Commission on Certification is only interested in the evaluation of the proposed contents. So what you are doing is killing two birds with one stone. You are being certified, and you are assisting in the development of the final certifying test that will be administered in July of 1975. Now if you are eligible and you do not offer your input, then you should not complain about the instrument that is finally developed. In effect, you are being asked to do an item analysis of the test so that poor items can be deleted and good items can be retained.

Counselor certification was an abstract concept just a few years ago. I've attended a number of national and regional meetings where they discussed this; it was very abstract, and most people thought the concept would never get off the ground. Let me tell you—it's real, and it's rapidly becoming an integral part of this field of rehabilitation. It's very possible, and this may sound funny, or you may say this is stupid, but it may be possible that counselor certification will be just as common as the R-4 in a few years and will become not only the norm but the expected. What I am saying is that whether you agree or disagree with counselor certification, it is, in fact, a reality. And just a personal note—I'm going to take the test. I was so busy trying to provide information to other people that I missed the deadline date for the test that was given July 19, but I am going to take the test because I personally experience a great deal of anxiety when I am tested. I would much rather be the tester than the testee, and I have been playing that role in the university setting. Maybe the very fact that I am in the university and in the classroom makes me even more anxious about being examined at this late date in my professional life, so I plan to take it. I feel that perhaps I might benefit by being involved with it.

Now I know that there are a lot of questions that you might have. Some of the problems that have developed have been over professional membership—do I have to be a member of a professional organization? The answer to that is yes, and some of you are going to be very angry about this. The professional organizations that are considered important would be the American Rehabilitation Counseling Association, the National Rehabilitation Counseling Association, and the American Psychological Association, Div. 20 and 17. I am sorry to report to you that, at this time, being a member of ASPD and VEWA is not sufficient. I disagree with that but that is beside the point. If you plan to take the exam you must be a member of either NRCA, ARCA, or APA.

Another question has been related to when and where the test will be given again. The test that was given July 1, 1974, required that your application be in by March, 1974, and some of you met that deadline. I failed to meet it. Applicants who wish to take the October 15, 1974, exam must have had an application in by July 1, 1974. The exam to be given March 22, 1975, will require the filing of an application by December 1, 1974. This is the one that in all probability you will take if you haven't gotten your application in by now and you desire to take the test. The last exam will be October 12, 1975, and your application will have to be in and accepted by July 1, 1975. The Commission has also stated that the first test that was given July 19th was given at 40 sites across the country. I believe it was given in Knoxville and also in Memphis. The Commission has stated that in the future the test will be given at any place at which 20 counselors can be gathered together; that is, counselors who have submitted their applications and whose applications have been approved. Therefore, the test will be given if you have 20 counselors who desire to take it.

A lot of people have complained about the cost of the examination. Many thought that the examination would require only $15, and they were a little astonished when they found out that the $15 covered only the processing of the initial application. In order to take the test one must pay an additional $30, making a total of $45. If you are interested, I can give you an item by item cost on where this money is going. For instance, your $15 application fee is for the processing of the application only. This includes printing of the application, postage (each application is sent out registered mail), secretarial costs, and cost of the follow-up on the vita. When you submit your application you are also required to submit a vita, and they have to follow up this vita information to make sure it is accurate. Following the receipt of the application and the vita, the credentials committee meets to review the application to determine whether or not you are eligible to take the examination. You might be interested to know that during the last meeting of the credentials committee there were 1800 applications, and it took two days to review all of these. Members of the credentials committee come from all over the country, and travel and lodging expenses probably account for the first $15. The $30 is for the cost of development and administration of the exam and support of the certification commission.

Development of the exam includes two different processes. Process number one is the contract to develop the test. This included the development of 750 items with five discrete forms, so we have five forms with approximately 150 items. When you take the test you will take only one of the five forms, so you'll only have 150 items. You will tentatively evaluate each item according to whether you think it is a good item or a poor item. Somebody else will take Form B and will do the same. Then, in the end, they'll make an item analysis and come up with the final test. It costs $15 to develop each item, and there are 750 items. Somebody had to write these items. These people had to be trained to write the items. Included in costs are editing, typing, proofing, development of the test booklet and instructional booklet, cost of developing the item, training people to write the item, and then screening, receiving, and processing the item. I could go on and on and tell you for instance that it costs $2.70 per candidate to provide feedback on the exam. Once you take the exam ,somebody must give you some feedback.

Let me mention one more thing that might be encouraging to you. In most professional organizations that have a certifying procedure it is necessary that you be recertified each year, which means you have to pay a recertification fee. Well, the Commission on Certification has stated that you will not have to pay a recertifying fee until after the first five years. If the Commission receives 4,000 candidates the first year, the cost of the test per unit will be $17.00. If they receive only 500 candidates the first year, the cost will be $44.00 per unit. Assume that the Commission receives enough units the first year to earn $13.00 per unit, then the total earnings will be 4,000 x $13.00=$52,000.00. On a five-year basis this will mean $10,000 to the commission per year for support. The Commission is front loading its cost so that counselors will not have to pay for recertification until after the first five years. After the first five years, the recertification fee will be approximately $10. Renewal will be based on your continued professional and educational development (including inservice training, enrollment in institutions of higher education for advanced training, and continued membership in professional organizations).

Individualized Written Programs

Each year a State Plan for Vocational Rehabilitation is rewritten setting forth priorities and basic positions of the agency. This year's program includes both the severely disabled and the lesser handicapped and places greater emphasis than ever upon job placement and job development.

The focus of this paper is on the new emphasis on client involvement. The Rehabilitation Act of 1973 includes in its provisions a requirement for an Individualized Written Plan. The Individual Rehabilitation Plan is a document to be developed together by the client and counselor. The client is a participant in making decisions concerning the type of services rendered and suitable vocational objectives.

One purpose of the plan is to insure that the rehabilitation process is a continuing type of action that the counselor and client have developed together. Verbatim directives of this section of the Vocational Rehabilitation Act are given. One of the main criticisms of rehabilitation services over the years has been the lack of documentation and case recording. Implementation of the regulations discussed here will improve the quality and quantity of services.

There has never been a time when rehabilitation has been on the threshold of such great opportunities and challenges than right now. But, after all, we have had fifty-four years to develop the program, so it's not new. There are not many public programs that can stand for fifty-four years and still come out with their basic concepts, philosophy, goals, and objectives still intact. Not many programs can get by without showing age in fifty-four years—certainly people can't. We might look back for a brief moment at our achievements in order to gain from experience and continue to chart new courses. Then, we can look forward to all of the challenging opportunities that confront us.

It seems to me that the most pressing priority for Vocational Rehabilitation is to demonstrate, as it has done in the past, that such a program can provide the basic framework for severely disabled people who may necessitate new directions, new procedures, and some new techniques. This basic framework includes the rewriting each year of a State Plan for Vocational Rehabilitation. Such a document will set forth the priorities and basic position the state agency here in Tennessee intends to take in order to meet the needs of those who are severely disabled. As has been indicated, Congress did not mean for us to ignore those people with lesser handicaps. The framework will include those persons with lesser handicaps as well as the severely disabled. In addition, this legislation will also emphasize job placement and job development as never before in order to create more employment opportunities for those people we serve. The job *is* the vocational aspect. There is also a need to place new emphasis on client participation in individualized written programs. This new emphasis presupposes more scrutiny of the vocational rehabilitation process because such participation has meant so much to so many people for so many years. I have no crystal ball to use here in the next few minutes, but I want to share some things about this program as I see it.

We now have many new mandates facing us, and I think we are equal to the challenge. The Rehabilitation Act of 1973 has many new and exciting provisions, many of which have been mentioned this morning. I wish to mention one or two before we finish. Some of these provisions seem to overshadow others because they were so much a part of what Congress was thinking when it drafted and passed this legislation. They dominated the discussions in Congressional hearings and reports and have consequently become the focus of our implementation activities. These are the mandates which influence and can be influenced by each one of us right here in this room.

Before discussing the Individualized Written Rehabilitation Program, there are a couple of things I would like to mention. One of the top priorities inherent in the Act is that vocation rehabilitation must give special attention to severely disabled people. The problems and/or disabilities of severely handicapped people are often so great that, in order to solve them, multiple services are needed over an extended period of time. In my opinion, everything we do must be weighed in relation to this objective. The sum of our efforts should show this group as our main target. This must be done, however, without sacrificing services and direction to those persons with lesser handicaps. Standards for operations, case services, and accountability must characterize the provisions for service in our program so they will be better understood by the public. In addition they should engender greater respect and responsiveness from the clientele that we serve. When we achieve our goals and objectives and report 400,000, 500,000, and 600,000 rehabilitations each year, then other agencies, organizations, and individuals will be made aware of the clients' need for the services of Vocational Rehabilitation. As we report our other program accomplishments, we will need to continue to be very conscious of our production goals. Much more could be said about the various aspects of Vocational Rehabilitation, but I would like now to discuss one very specific phase of our program: the new emphasis on client involvement.

Greater stress must be placed on client participation in the Vocational Rehabilitation process, in addition to improved case services to handicapped individuals and their families. The Individualized Rehabilitation Plan is an important document. It is a plan to be developed by the client and the counselor together. Regardless of how this specific provision became law, we must accept it. This relationship between client and counselor is the key to the way our work is done. For the past several years a great deal more attention has been given to client participation (even without legislation). Client needs have been reflected not only in terms of vocational opportunities, but also in terms of transportation and housing. Problems for severely disabled people in these areas often appear insurmountable. For instance, what are the problems for a wheelchair case or a double brace, double crutch, or blind person in trying to ride a bus or attempting to get from home to the job?

The Rehabilitation Act of 1973 mandates important new directions and services to the handicapped to overcome many of these barriers and problems. This Act established a partnership between the recipient, the agency, and the counselor who represents the recipient. For perhaps the first time the client becomes a participant, an equal partner in making the decisions which will help in meeting his individual needs—decisions concerning the type of services rendered and suitable vocational objectives to be achieved. Providing the client with information upon which certain determinations can be made is an important function of the agency representative. This Act provides for the protection of the rights of the recipients. Most importantly, it provides for participation of the client in determining the kind of services that are needed. These decisions should be based on what counselors have talked with him about, have interpreted to him, and have helped him understand about himself from the beginning. In many situations, after services have been completed and employment secured, the counselor-client relationship continues to be supportive in nature, and thereby the rehabilitant has the assurances of the continued support of the counselor and the agency as may be appropriate to his particular case.

I was a rehabilitation counselor for a number of years, and I am very proud of this opportunity I had to help people move along the continuum we call the rehabilitation process. This continuum generally follows the line of case finding, evaluation, planning, services, placement, and follow-up. In order to do this, we had a document called a Rehabilitation Plan which was implemented in 1944, possibly prior to that date in some other states. This plan was called the R-5, the Rehabilitation Plan, and to some degree it was developed jointly. It required that the client and I both sign this plan. On the form I had to report such items of information as the client's name, vocational objectives, disability, age, and kind of services we planned (we, meaning the client and myself) and agreed were needed in order to solve identified problems and barriers such as unemployment or impending unemployment if problems were not solved. The counselor told the client about the type of services, costs involved, and when they were going to start and hopefully when these services would end, and what benefits would likely accrue. We also tried to include justification for the job objective that had been chosen as well as justification for the kind of services rendered. We were working with public funds and were required to justify how we arrived at particular services or job objectives. All of the states had a similar type of plan. This was thirty years ago, so why would we at this point in the development of vocational rehabilitation still be talking about that aspect of rehabilitation to the extent of including a written individualized program into the Act itself?

Section 101 of the Act (P.L. 93-112) referred to this point and provided that a state agency will have this kind of form. In Section 102, a detailed listing of what was included in the plan was given. Some of the items included in this Section were mentioned earlier. So, it's in the Act. It's also in the Regulations. Section 401.38 deals with a kind of blown-up version. It simply lists all these provisions for the Individualized Written Plan or program for the client, lifted right out of the Act, and it doesn't really matter at this point whether the Regulations have been approved or not because the same Provision is in the Act. The Act has been signed and is in the process of being implemented. Therefore, the Provision is with us to stay. The underlying purpose of having the Written Individualized Program within the Act and Regulations is to provide better continuity as well as more participation of the client in his own rehabilitation.

We talked about the rehabilitation process as a continuum of services, starting with case finding, evaluating, planning, providing services, placement, and follow-up. One purpose of the Plan is to give more continuity to make sure that the rehabilitation process is a continuing type of activity that the counselor and the client have developed together. It presupposes that pertinent data and information have been pooled about the client, information that will be useful in finding solutions to individual problems. The rehabilitation process provides a chance to plan together, make decisions jointly, and develop better case management.

Now, what about the timing? The Act says that a written program is required concurrent with or reasonably soon after the Certificate of Eligibility is given. As soon as the Certificate is executed or the plan made for evaluation, the written program must be developed before the initiation of services. However, services may be started on the basis of interim programs if such is in the interest of the client. If this interim program is developed jointly with the client, it should include a specific date by which the regular program will be developed. The basic program should be understood as being a starting point and subject to additions, changes, supplements, and amendments. All subsequent entries must be dated, too. Congress certainly specified continuity within the Act to eliminate long unexplained gaps that one sees from time to time in some case records.

As the plan is being developed between client and counselor, more information is accumulated and evaluated. There is an awareness that a plan is being created according to a mutual decision making process. Typically, this activity is recorded in the case file where the program is formally written by the counselor for the case records. The Written Individualized Plan is a synthesis of what has taken place. As counselors gather information, they sometimes get more than can be used. Thus, it is the counselor's responsibility to ferret out or differentiate significant facts from those that are insignificant or do not have a bearing on the rehabilitation program that is being developed. All pertinent information must be included.

In summary, I have lifted almost verbatim from the Vocational Rehabilitation Act of 1973, Public Law 93-112, and I will read from the Section of the Regulations, Section 401.38, Individualized Written Rehabilitation Program. I will try to lay out the main facts in each of these since there are at least fifteen items here that will summarize what I have been saying:

The Individualized Written Rehabilitation Programs shall contain all relevant information about the individual and the services provided. The individualized written program shall include, but not necessarily be limited to, data supporting the following: (1) the determination of eligibility or ineligibility or the decision to put the person in extended evaluation; (2) the written individualized rehabilitation program shall support any determination that the handicapped individual is severely handicapped; (3) it shall also support the determination of the vocational rehabilitation services to be provided and the terms and conditions for the provision of such services including in the event that physical and mental restoration services are provided and the determination that the clinical status of the client's disabling condition is stable or slowly progressive; (4) the projected date for the initiation of each vocational rehabilitation service, the anticipated duration of each service and the time within which the objectives and goals for each individual may be achieved; (5) a procedure and schedule for evaluation of the progress made by the person reaching the rehabilitation goal; (6) a long-range employment goal for the individual as well as the intermediate ones that will have to be taken into consideration; (7) it shall also give assurances that the handicapped individual has been informed of his rights and the means by which he may express and seek remedy for his dissatisfaction, including opportunities for administrative reviews and a fair hearing; and (8) an assurance that the handicapped individual has been advised about the confidentiality of all the information which he and his counselor have accumulated with respect to his situation: medical information, psychiatric information, vocational information, social information, making sure that he or she understands that this is strictly professional and confidential.

The only reason we get the data and the only reason we probe so much is because we think the information will have a bearing on the vocational objective selected for the individual as well as the kinds of services that will be needed. It will also help the agency representative establish eligibility. There are several other items included, but I think we have covered the main points. Now what kind of format will be used or developed? I suspect that many state agencies have already developed or experimented with a form that will suffice.

As was indicated this morning, it will take more manpower to further implement this plan. One of the criticisms of rehabilitation over the years has been the lack of documentation and case recording. We have done many reviews from time to time in federal offices for the primary purpose of trying to help state agencies improve the quality and quantity of services. Many times we have discovered a very inadequate case recording system. I suspect that state agencies will want to begin to implement this particular provision even though it will probably prove to be a bit burdensome in the beginning. I suggest that you study very carefully all of the items in Section 401.38 of the Regulations because I have not had time to include all of the provisions here. You may also want to study Section 102 of Public Law 93-112, which specifies all of the requirements for the Individualized Written Rehabilitation Program in detail.

Placement of the Severely Disabled

The ultimate objective of the rehabilitation counselor is to help the disabled find work. Too often the client comes with little work experience and has never experienced success and achievment in work. To find ways and means of integrating the severely disabled into the world of work will require finding and utilizing all available resources and will require the integrity and commitment of all professionals dealing with the client.

Utilization of the whole community is necessary for optimum service to the severely disabled. The community can best respond when it understands the objectives of the program and understands that it is needed.

The rehabilitation counselor grows in creativity, versatility, adaptability, and resourcefulness, plus many more intangible qualities as he deals with clients, with prejudice, and with the social environment. He attempts to open doors of opportunity for the severely disabled to be able to change, grow, and develop into productive wage earners.

Thinking in terms of basic human needs is the key to working effectively with and through other people. Recognition and nourishment of needs in other than the severely disabled can be the way to reach those in the community who can be of help. Examples of implementation of these operational principles aid in understanding the concept of "people" factors.

As the years have come and gone and as I've dealt with a number of generations of students at Oklahoma State University, I sometimes wonder how in the world anyone would ever have the temerity or the daring to put himself in a position where he attempts to help another person in a way that makes a real difference. Consider this question: Can we even begin to imagine all the things we should have by way of background and understanding and empathy and warmth and genuineness and knowledge? An even more sobering thought is that we are here to consider ways of positively helping those who are considered "severely disabled."

Who are the severely disabled? I have no cut and dried definition. In my work as a rehabilitation counselor I have often found that some of the people who, according to all the classifications were the most severely disabled, really were much less severely disabled than some of the other people who, according to the literal classifica-

37

tions, were marginal. Now I won't quibble over the particulars. Even though we do have some realistic kinds of bench marks, disability is a relative kind of thing. I recall being at a National Rehabilitation Association Conference in Miami Beach, Florida, several years ago and drifting down the beach one day for lunch. The restaurant was crowded. Seated directly across from me was a man who quite obviously was in the later stages of Parkinson's disease. I glanced at this man, and he looked across at me. He locked his gaze on my balding head. Finally in a tone bordering on pity he asked me, "Tell me, mister, how in the world did you ever lose your hair?" So I guess that when we come to the matter of defining the severely disabled we will continue to find differences of opinion.

Before I launch into what I hope will become provocative thoughts, I want to tell you that I do not come here with a neat bag of tricks. I've been in the business too long. And regardless of what I say or how I might sound as I get wound up on a point or two, I realize that you and I are in a field where failure is not uncommon. I do not, by any means, have insight into ways and means that for any one particular individual will absolutely guarantee success. My experience has taught me to be highly suspicious of anyone who suggests this. At the same time I am hoping to share some ideas that have come to me in ways that will help us to glimpse another angle or some guiding principle or some concept that will assist us as we go about meeting the challenge that now has been mandated by legislation: finding ways and means of integrating into the mainstream of society people who are identified as severely disabled.

Our ultimate objective is to help them find one of the most desirable things in all the world—*work*. About all it takes is for a person to be incapacitated for one day to realize what a tremendous privilege the ability to work is. How great it is to return to the job after being sick! How deeply do we feel it is the right of our severely handicapped citizens to experience the meaning of productive activity? Too often these people come to us with a lack of work experience. Many have not been habilitated, much less rehabilitated. In some cases they don't want to work. But it would appear that more often through experiencing a lack of success and lack of achievement they have had to come to terms with life in ways that, being denied the opportunity to work, often forced them to find satisfaction in other ways.

Recently I came across an article called "What Size Is a Dream?" I was reminded of this as I looked out over the Mississippi River this afternoon. I suddenly connected what I am trying to get across to you with the need for a river bridge. My mind went back to early times, the pioneering days, when the settlers were faced with trying to cross the Mississippi River. It was an "impossible" task, wasn't it? The analogy came to my mind that in many respects the segment of the population you and I are attempting to place can be compared to pioneers beating their way through the wilderness and trying to cross the Mississippi without a bridge.

As I mused on the analogy my thoughts retreated in history to the early 1800's when President Jefferson commissioned a couple of fellows by the name of Lewis and Clark to survey the immense territory called the Louisiana Purchase. It was an "impossible" task, wasn't it? Perhaps it really would have been an impossible task if they had relied on doing it all by themselves. You want to know how they did it? Go buy a copy of the paperback edition of the abridged journals of Lewis and Clark. You will find it fascinating. You will also quickly see the analogy between those leaders approaching their task and us as we carry out our charge to explore and develop a new kind of Louisiana Purchase.

When reading the journal of Lewis and Clark you learn that before they took one step in the direction of the Pacific Coast they engaged in a fantastic amount of preparation. It is almost unbelievable to read of the extent to which they availed themselves of all the essential resources as they looked toward the great unknown—crossing an unexplored continent. It was not easy. What size is a dream? And what is involved in making a dream a reality? How big is our dream? And what is involved in making a dream a reality? How big is our dream of being able to place the severely handicapped? It depends on those doing the dreaming, doesn't it? and on how much they really believe in what they are doing—on how much preparation they are willing to make. For some a dream can expand to infinity—sparked with colors, possibilities, and new vistas. For others it may be a longing for a decent job, a new suit of clothes, and plenty of warm food to eat.

Too often the person who has been classified as severely disabled or severely handicapped is not allowed to scale the wall into the bigger world. And my question is simply, "Why not?" Why is it necessary for us to mount an offensive, as it were, a Lewis and Clark expedition of sorts, to explore the wilderness, to find ways and means of integrating the severely disabled into the world of work? What's keeping them from being productive? What's keeping employers from hiring them? When you ask such questions you begin to wonder all over again just how much "stick-to-it-iveness" we have. How courageous are we? How willing are we to be champions for those who are denied the chance to do what they are able to do? We must be a strange breed of cat in order to really believe in what it is we are talking about. I had the privilege not long ago of speaking to a group of people in Dallas who work with the deaf-blind. I am reminded of some thoughts I brought to their attention which I would also like to share with you.

Ultimately the utilization of our assets, no matter how well endowed we are with facilities or funds or know-how, will be at the mercy of the integrity and commitment of the professionals who interpret and deliver the services on the firing line. The success or failure of any major effort to rehabilitate those called "severely disabled" will depend on human variables operating in each of us. If we were so disposed, you and I could fill these walls with dozens—even hundreds—of reasons why we cannot succeed. The chances are that in many instances the clients themselves would believe it. Rather than think in terms of being made part of a productive work force, we can prove to them that it is better to go some other route. Believe me, you will not have too much trouble proving to the man on the street today that rehabilitation of the severely disabled can't be done. We can give up a thousand times, and few will castigate us; we can throw in the towel and people will say we finally saw the light.

Why would even seasoned professionals sometimes shy away from tackling the multi-faceted problems inherent in trying to place the severely handicapped? Could it be that we have failed even to dimly glimpse the range of human potential? Research has shown that most of us use only 10-25 per cent of what the Good Lord gave us as our birthright. No wonder, with such a litmited understanding and self-development, the larger society tends to classify the severely handicapped as "hopeless."

We are born with 10,000, 000,000 brain cells, each with up to 60,000 junction points, whose interplay has eluded the best minds.

It seems that the majority of the brain cells of mankind are doomed to remain in eternal infancy.

How alert are we? How alive are we? Experiments have shown that many sighted people may come and go in a particular room for years—and yet when given a test it is shown that they actually have never looked at the room. How many windows are there? What is the color of the trim around the doors? What is the location of the fire extinguisher? This is a simple example of the kind of self-inflicted no man's land we inhabit when it would require little additional effort to come alive, really come alive.

I have an almost childlike faith in man and what he can become. That is idealism, and I want to keep it forever. At the same time I deal with the reality of people where they are. Consequently I am seldom surprised no matter what happens.

This is being a kind of professional schizophrenic. It requires living on a unique sort of intrinsic motivation. Like Job of old, our friends can certainly question our sanity when we persist for one year, two years, or X years in pursuing our objectives with little assurance that we will be "successful" in the popular sense of the word, yet we dare to be in business—and stay in business. We work both for short-range and long-range goals. We live and thrive on secondary satisfactions. Even witnessing to a minor degree tiny evidences of self-discovery and growth in one of our clients is to revive and renew our feeling of enthusiasm and belief in the value of our cause. We refuse to be detered by disappointment. There must be some way!

Let us use another analogy. The Koala bear refuses to eat anything but eucalyptus leaves. And of all the varieties of eucalyptus, the Koala will eat leaves from but *one* variety. He knows the way, you see. Contrast the Koala with the coyote. The coyote is cunning, adaptable, resourceful, ever alert for ways of using his surrounding environment to aid in the achievement of his objectives. To my mind, the outstanding professional who proposes to find ways to discover and use resources in his environment to help place the severely handicapped is a coyote of sorts. If the idea of comparing yourself to a coyote is distasteful, then identify with someone or something which to you represents the epitome of creativity and versatility.

Actually I resist the idea of using the term "severely handicapped." Words are one of the most useful of all discoveries, but they can have a deadening, stereotyping effect. To a significant degree we are struggling to overcome much more than the effects of severely handicapping conditions per se. We are faced with the much more elusive and insidious enemy of "labelitis." We must be extremely careful in our choice of words as we attempt to open doors of opportunity. We know full well that the population labeled as the severely handicapped can be rehabilitated; that is, if and when we can overcome a major barrier in the "deafness" and "blindness" of those who let labels immobilize any concept of such people being able to change, grow, and develop into productive wage earners.

Patience is the hallmark of the professional in this field. We live on the verge of another tiny breakthrough which could come at any time. Minor successes sustain and nourish the excitement of the pioneer who knows that the unexplored spaces of a human being contain treasures and riches untold if they can but be discovered and developed.

Ultimately all the resources of the agency are at the mercy of intangible but very real human resources. These include the vision, the imagination, the intelligence, the patience, the philosophy, the skills, the understanding, the resourcefulness, the integrity of character, the enthusiasm, the courage, the diplomacy, and the judgment of everyone across the board who influences in any way the policies of an agency and the provision of services which culminate in placement.

The quality of these fragile and variable human resources determines decisions that can figuratively open or close the door of opportunity for a handicapped person. Such concepts and factors as "feasibility," how much the family will be involved, the degree and ways in which a diversity of community resources will be utilized, and the breadth and depth of placement exploration—all of these and many more considerations are subject to decisions of the professional. What a responsibility!

The larger community must be utilized if we are to get the job done. The understanding and philosophy of the professional person, to be truly effective, must come alive in the hands and feet and brains of the employers, the attitude and understanding of the larger community, and the attitude and understanding of the client and his family. In order for Lewis and Clark to reach the mouth of the Columbia River, they had to work with and through other people. Without the Indian lady, Sacajawea, and friendly Indian tribes, they would never have made it to the Pacific Northwest. They were masters in the art and science of public relations. Things did not happen simply because they had good intentions. The native Americans responded when they understood the objectives of the expedition, when they understood they were needed, and when they were treated with respect.

What are some ways we can work effectively with and through other people in order to give our clientele an opportunity to earn their livings? I think part of the answer is probably so obvious that we sometimes have passed it by. I challenge you to think in terms of basic human needs. I come back to this theme time and again as I deal with students. Let us identify some of these needs: the need for acceptance, shelter and security; the need for achievement, other people and recognition; and the need for appreciation, communication and discovery.

Let me at this point state that we realize a business must make a profit. We also need to point out that if we have done our homework before approaching an employer we are convinced our client will make a profit for the employer. We have evaluated, diagnosed and counseled the client. We have studied the client. We know his assets and his liabilities. We are aware of what, if any, specialized supervision may be needed. With these assumptions made, let us proceed to the "people" factors.

There is a master keyboard in every individual. The profit motive is a big key to the employer, but there are many other keys on his "needs" keyboard. An employer is, first of all, a person, isn't he? As such, he yearns for recognition. He needs to be involved and feel needed. He is often searching for more meaning and reason for being. Why can't these keys be "tapped" in appropriate ways which will work to the advantage and satisfaction of both the employer and the client? For example, it is unbelievable what one will do if you develop a symbol, a plaque, a certificate that respects achievement and recognition in the eyes of a person's peers. The Employer of the Year award at whatever level—local, state, or national—is but one legitimate way we can utilize the recognition and nourishment of needs in others.

Let us take another example. Several years ago I had a student complete an assignment which called for identifying innovative or different ways of using resources on behalf of the handicapped. This fellow came up with the idea of annually having a "Taxi Driver of the Year" award for the taxi driver who had been most outstanding in helping place the handicapped. Again I am referring to the master keyboard. I'm speaking about our understanding of the human nature of human beings. People are first of all people. Before taxi drivers are taxi drivers they are people; before a doctor is a doctor he's a "people"; before a counselor is a counselor he or she is "people." In varying degrees each one of us needs the kind of nourishment that comes through these factors that we mentioned. Constructively, creatively, we can use the concepts of recognition, of appreciation, of achievement in ways that will help us build that Mississippi River bridge. Lewis and Clark got to the West Coast by working with and through other people, and they did it not by withdrawing from basic human needs of the native Americans, but by taking them into account.

People want to help. We need their help. With our assistance they can come to a much better understanding of our cause and philosophy. Through selective screening and education of others we can multiply many times what one person can do. And if we find sincere, genuine and visible means of recognizing their efforts—of making them feel more worthwhile to themselves and their peers— we will have an inexhaustible gold mine of resources.

We must look at and combine the common in an uncommon way.

I believe that the rehabilitation professional, as he deals with clients, as he deals with prejudice, as he tries, as it were, to tackle the matter of surveying the Louisiana Purchase of the severely disabled, develops out of necessity a kind of extended vision, an alertness, a diversity of ways of looking at things. And I'm not trying to make anyone a superman or a superwoman. I'm talking about the person who really begins to utilize in a major way the great potential I mentioned earlier. I refer to this in some respects as an "A.Q." You've heard of an I.Q. "A.Q." is what I call an "Awareness Quotient." Just how sensitive are we? How aware are we of the world around us?

Some of you in this room either have known personally or know by reputation the fellow who was my state director when I was a rehabilitation counselor. His name is J. J. Brown. Anything, literally anything, that people do is of interest to Mr. Brown. If you are following Mr. Brown in a car, you dare not follow too closely, for if he happens to glance over the countryside and notes anyone doing something that to him is "different," he will more than likely come to a screeching halt. He has an urge to investigate, to discuss and to know.

Mr. Brown not only is a big man physically. He has a mental stomach which has an enormous capacity. He is forever asking questions. He samples and savors the things which occur in the course of everyday life. When he was a state rehabilitation director, he actively sought new experiences. He connected names with faces, and he cared enough to remember.

Using another analogy, the person skilled in placement is a kind of Sherlock Holmes who finds literally dozens of leads for ways to exploit the social environment for a possible job placement. Such an individual views with great interest the construction of an apartment house or a new hotel or an industrial park or a new hospital. He sees past the outline of concrete and steel and envisions all the different activities and the people needed to carry out those activities. He can see dozens of hundreds of people performing a wide variety of jobs. He sees custodians, maintenance personnel, receptionists, secretaries, messengers, apprentices, executives, foremen. He not only sees the pattern of a mosaic of people and buildings present and projected, but he also studies each part of the pattern and how it relates to all the rest.

It requires this kind of individual to bring to life the thing we call serendipity. Another word for serendipity is "the Happy Accident." A closer look at what usually takes place reveals that it is not an "accident" at all. Rather, the individual has so immersed himself in a given area that he is much more sensitive to and alert for clues which others usually pass by. I am reminded of one of our graduates, James Dixon, who is an avid fisherman. Mr. Dixon can be driving along the road and pick up clear indications of there being a farm pond or a good fishing place nearby while others in the same car viewing the same landscape see few such indications.

We are speaking of seeing with an inner eye—of listening with a third ear. We think of people as exciting untapped resources. We not only think of who, but we think of what? how? where? when? We consider different combinations of these alternatives. We stay eternally alert for the flash of insight, the germ of an idea, or the suggestion that may be picked up from a peer. We get in groups such as this, and we brainstorm with one another. We exchange ideas; we build on ideas; we combine ideas. Even though we may have come fresh from failure on a previous case, we keep drawing sustenance from the basic philosophy that our failure did not necessarily prove it couldn't be done. On the contrary, while no one expects to have a 1.000 batting average, we can tolerate the suspicion that maybe, just maybe, we didn't find the right combination; we did not press the right buttons. Who knows? Maybe tomorrow we shall!

I have not attempted to outline to you a comprehensive how-to-do-it plan. Rather I have shared several basic concepts which I trust will stimulate us to take a fresh look at how we see ourselves, our clients, and others. Too, I have shared some operational principles which I suggest we seriously consider as we attempt to find and implement better ways of placing our brothers and sisters who are severely handicapped.

Carl E. Hansen

Rehabilitation Counselor Certification

After clarification of the differences between accreditation and certification, reasons for establishing counselor certification procedures are given. Important points are that such certification would upgrade services to clients and that professional identity and independence would be fostered.

Details are given as to the actual mechanics of implementation of the program for certification, the way in which it is developed, a breakdown of the costs, and the reasons for the "grandfathering" period. Standards and criteria for certification are given in detail as well as the probable impact and implications of counselor certification.

As an introduction to this discussion, it is important to note that two concepts stand separate. The first concept is that certification is not synonymous with the National Rehabilitation Counseling Association. The National Rehabilitation Counseling Association had a great deal to do with the start and continued movement of the certification process, but it is not a part of the membership rights and privileges of the NRCA. Because one is a member of NRCA does not automatically mean that he is a certified rehabilitation counselor.

The second concept to keep in mind is that certification and accreditation are two very different terms and apply to two very different situations. Accreditation is a term reserved for rehabilitation counselor programs, whereas certification is a term reserved for the review and approval of the ability that an individual counselor exhibits. Certification applies to individuals; accreditation applies to training programs.

BASIC QUESTIONS

Throughout the last few years, many rehabilitation counselors have brought forward reasons why they feel certification is important. A brief review of these reasons should give the reader a greater understanding about why certification exists and why it is important for the field of rehabilitation counseling.

1. For many counselors certification appears to answer the question of establishing a minimum level of competency so that clients are assured basic services. It is felt that in time certification could eliminate questionable personnel; for example, personnel who do not have the appropriate background or abilities in the area of rehabilitation counseling to be working with disabled clients. This first reason is an extremely important one because it is based on a competency issue. It is the feeling of many people in rehabilitation that a basic level of competency must be met by each and every rehabilitation counselor before he be allowed to work with disabled clients.

2. Many rehabilitation counselors are concerned with professional identity and status. "Who are we? What are we really doing?" These two questions seem to stand important in many counselors' minds. It is felt that through certification, wherein a basic level of expertise would be developed, the professional identity of the rehabilitation counselor could be better identified.

3. It is felt by many counselors that certification will be imposed upon them by some other group if they do not certify themselves. Examples are given throughout the country wherein state legislatures have proposed placing rehabilitation counselors under the supervision of psychologists since psychologists have a certification and/or licensing structure. It is the feeling of certain state legislative bodies that the rehabilitation counselor is not a recognized professional identity and he should be placed under the supervision of a recognized professional. In one state it was suggested that the rehabilitation counselor work under the supervision of a social worker. The social work profession is recognized with its MSW and certification procedure, and therefore it seemed only appropriate in the minds of certain legislative representatives within that particular state that rehabilitation counselors be placed under the supervision of a social worker. This very vividly points out that the rehabilitation counselor has a problem regarding professional status and that, if the counselor does not move toward a certifying position, then his role and function may be subsumed under a professional group that is recognized by certification.

4. Greater strength in vying for salary, vacation time, and benefits in general is felt by some counselors as a strength found in certification. This argument may weaken the certification procedure, but on the other hand this may be the way to stem the growing tide toward unionism. The utilization of certification, a bringing together of counselors with similar backgrounds and similar goals, could help team the tide of union membership. Certification is usually identified with high professional issues, but in this instance it is felt by many rehabilitation counselors that identity for the purposes of personal benefits for the rehabilitation counselor could be better attained if certification were to become a reality.

5. Many state agency rehabilitation counselors purchase services from facilities rendered to them by individuals called rehabilitation counselors. It is felt by many counselors that individuals working within facilities should meet some type of minimal competency base.

6. Rehabilitation counseling in the private domain would be better controlled if certification were brought about. Although there are few places in the United States where rehabilitation counselors enter private practice, it does hold potential for the future. It would be important for the disabled individual who may be purchasing his own service from a rehabilitation counselor that he be counseled by a person having a minimal degree of competency.

7. Many rehabilitation counselors throughout the country see the importance of certification for rehabilitation counselors as they view other fields that have certified professionals. Probably one of the most unique examples came from a rehabilitation counselor who wondered, since automobile mechanics in certain states had to go through a certification procedure, why rehabilitation counselors didn't? Wasn't it just as important to have competent individuals working with disabled citizens as it was to have competent individuals working as automobile mechanics?

In summary, these points seem to set the stage for the reasons many rehabilitation counselors desire certification. The key issues seem to be in two specific areas. The first area that is important, and that the majority of rehabilitation counselors who push for certification seem most concerned with, is the upgrading of services to clients by making sure that the rehabilitation counselor has a basic degree of competency.

The second point that seems key and important in this discussion is that certification can foster professional independency and identity. Professional independency and a professional identity may become more important as rehabilitation counselors become more involved with legislative funding issues. The last couple of years has seen rehabilitation encounter difficulties with the federal Congress in passing legislation and appropriations. If the field of rehabilitation counseling is to demonstrate that it has the maturity and ability to work with severely disabled clients and to conduct a program spending millions and millions of dollars, it must have a body of workers who have reached a degree of professional competency that ensures the general public that tax dollars are being well spent. These two points seem key in any discussion concerning reasons why certification should come about for the rehabilitation counselor.

REHABILITATION CERTIFICATION COMMISSION

As previously described, the Certification Commission is an independent body composed in membership of professional organizations and representative rehabilitation personnel and organizations. The National Rehabilitation Counseling Association appointed five members to this Commission. The American Rehabilitation Counseling Association appointed five members to this Commission. Commission members were also drawn from the Council of State Administrators for Vocational Rehabilitation. Medical, consumer, and education groups are represented; non-white and consumer representatives are included; and there is a representative from rehabilitation facilities. This fifteen-man Commission has as its president Dr. Dan McAlees, who is the Dean of the School of Rehabilitation and Special Education at the University of Northern Colorado, Greeley, Colorado.

The Commission decides all policy pertaining to the certification of rehabilitation counselors. No single commission composed of voluntary membership, though, is able to conduct and implement a program of certification that would be on a nation-wide scale. One of the first actions necessary for the Certification Commission was to draw up a set of guidelines for the bidding and ultimate acceptance of a company that could implement a certification program. There was interest shown from the University of Wisconsin, a testing firm in North Carolina, the Professional Examination Service, and NAT Resources, Ultimately, the Commission decided that NAT Resources, a Chicago-based firm, would be the most appropriate firm to conduct the actual mechanics of certification. NAT Resources is an established firm that has been working in the health and allied professions conducting certification programs for medical specialties for a number of years.

PROCEDURE AND COSTS

At the present time it takes $15 to apply for certification and an additional $30 at the time the certification test is taken. This totals $45. Many rehabilitation counselors are concerned that the cost is prohibitive and are concerned that too much money is being spent for the certification procedure. If we look at these costs, a number of factors evolve that describe and define where the money is being spent. First of all, test sites must be provided throughout the United States, and to set these up and to have monitors and proctors available during the tests is an expensive procedure. Additional costs are now being generated since a test site will be set up at any place where twenty rehabilitation counselors are available and desire to take the certification examination. This means that, in addition to the usual test centers throughout the United States, additional sites will be set up to meet the needs of counselors. During the 1974-75 year, five tests will be conducted.

Test sites and the arrangement for such testing and the proctoring of such examinations are only small factors involved in the cost. The sheer handling of the mail volume is an expensive procedure. Staff must be available to respond to questions pertaining to the certification procedure, handle applications and then check to see that the applications have been completed in the appropriate manner, guarantee that those individuals applying for certification meet the basic qualifications, and correspond with each applicant to let him know where the test site will be, when the test will be given, and so forth. This type of secretarial management is expensive, particularly since no one guessed that the number of applicants would be as high as they are now.

The development of the test alone is an expensive procedure.

No single individual can sit down and design a test that will be appropriate to the field of rehabilitation counseling. The Certification Commission very wisely decided first of all to organize a task force to study techniques in certification procedures and to invite this task force for a meeting so that all of its members could write questions that would be appropriate to the field of rehabilitation counseling. The task force was composed of counselors, educators, and supervisory personnel from throughout the United States. This particular task force had to submit questions that had to be reviewed by employed staff to see that they met the design of correct testing procedures. The task force will have to meet routinely to see that the test questions have a sound base and are being utilized appropriately on the testing instrument. Maintaining a confidential bank on current computer technology is an important issue. The company selected for the certification program had to have a computer output and ability that would maintain for each individual applying for certification a confidential record of his application and the results of his examination.

Costs are involved in developing equal but multiple forms of the test. A single test would not be adequate to meet the needs of the rehabilitation counseling certification movement. Multiple forms of the test must be developed and multiple forms must be equal in their strength in determining the knowledge of the rehabilitation counselor. This means that individuals with statistical ability and testing background must be employed to develop multiple forms of the test. Along this same line of thinking, there must be a thorough review of each item and its total contribution to the test. Each item must be statistically reviewed to see whether it has the strength to stay in a complete bank of questions. The test items must be reviewed to see if they are penalizing certain individuals. The question of minorities being penalized is certainly an issue, but a larger issue may be that of whether or not the test discriminates in favor of the state rehabilitation counselor as opposed to the private agency rehabilitation counselor. It is important that a thorough review be undertaken and an analysis be complete so that questions are appropriate to the state agency and the private agency rehabilitation counselor alike. There develops also a problem of appropriate examination procedures for those counselors who carry highly specialized caseloads of clients, such as the mentally retarded, the severely physically disabled, the epileptic, and so forth. It could very well be found through analysis that certain sub-tests will have to be developed for those counselors who carry specialized caseloads. This may mean that a core of questions will be given to all individuals applying for certification as a rehabilitation counselor, and then certain specialty sub-tests might be given to those individuals who are carrying a highly specialized caseload.

During 1974-75 a "grandfathering" period of time is being made available to analyze and test the certification procedure. During the twelve-month years from July 1, 1974, through July 1, 1975, the testing procedure will be examined, and those individuals who are applying for certification who meet all qualifications will have to take the test as a standardizing procedure. They will not have to pass the test with any type of cutoff score. Only those taking the test after July 1, 1975, will have to reach a minimum cutoff score to be considered certified rehabilitation counselors. The "grandfathering" period of time is extremely important in that it allows the Certification Commission and the company handling certification a period of time in which to evaluate their items from a statistical and normative standpoint so that the test will be appropriate to the needs of the field during the period of time following the "grandfathering" era.

STANDARDS AND CRITERIA FOR REHABILITATION COUNSELOR CERTIFICATION

Professional rehabilitation counselor certification may be established by:

1. Graduation with a master's degree from an accredited rehabilitation counseling training program that includes a supervised internship, the completion of which ensures minimum content acquisition as specified, and one year of acceptable experience* in rehabilitation counseling.

---

*Acceptable experience in rehabilitation counseling is defined as full-time employment acceptable to the Commission in the use of rehabilitative counseling techniques; vocational evaluation; psychological assessment; social, medical, and vocational psychiatric information; and rehabilitative methods in an agency (public or private), hospital or clinic, in which the applicant is under professional supervision and has employed such methods and measures. By 1977, acceptable experience will require supervision by a person certified in rehabilitation counseling by the National Commission on Rehabilitaton Counselor Certfication.

2. Attainment of a master's degree in rehabilitation counseling, not including a supervised internship, or a master's degree in a related area (as defined by the Commission), along with two years of experience in rehabilitation counseling and competence in the content areas specified below.
3. Attainment of a master's degree equivalency level by one of the following:
   a. Graduation with a bachelor's degree in rehabilitation along with four years of acceptable experience in rehabilitation counseling and competence in the content areas specified be-below.
   b. Graduation with a bachelor's degree along with five years of acceptable experience in rehabilitation counseling and competence in the content specified below.
4. Demonstration of competence in the following content areas:
   a. Rehabilitation philosophy, history, and structure
   b. Medical aspects of disability
   c. Psycho-social aspects of handicapped conditions
   d. Occupational information and the world of work
   e. Counseling theory and techniques
   f. Community organization and resources
   g. Placement processes and job development
   h. The psychology of personal and vocational adjustment
   i. Evaluation and assessment
   j. The ability to utilize research findings and professional publications.

"Grandfathering" those members who meet the above criteria will be carried out by July, 1975, according to the time schedule established by the National Commission on Rehabilitation Counselor Certification. After that date all persons who qualify for certification will be required to pass a certification examination. Membership in ARCA, NRCA, and/or an allied professional association will be a prerequisite for "grandfathering."

For those not meeting the above criteria, an applicant who deems himself qualified to be a rehabilitation counselor and has five years of experience or its equivalent may apply to the National Commission and, at the discretion of the Credentials Committee, may take the examination to be "grandfathered."

During the "grandfathering" period, all applicants meeting the criteria of the Commission will be required to take the certification examination, but will not be required to achieve a minimum specified score.

WILL IT BE WORTH IT?

We know at the present time that it costs a total of $45 to register and take the certification test. It is significant to note that the certification movement has been totally sponsored by the field. Two years ago many rehabilitation counselors voluntarily contributed money to get the certification movement started, and now each individual is voluntarily paying a minimum of $45 to have certification become an individual reality. This is compared to the accreditation movement which has cost thousands and thousands of dollars through a Rehabilitation Service Administration grant so that the accreditation of university programs could move toward reality. The individual-counselor certification has not cost the taxpayers a single dollar. At the present time, in August, 1974, over 3,000 individuals have signed up to take the certification examination. This number exceeds all expectations, particularly at such an early date in the "grandfathering" period.

The basic question, though, "Will it be worth $45?" must be seriously considered. This question can be reviewed from three standpoints: first, for the disabled client it would appear that to establish a base of competency so that the disabled client in America is assured that he will have systematic and competent individuals working with him is most assuredly worth $45.

Second, for the facility and private rehabilitation counselor it would appear to be worth it. Facility and private rehabilitation counselors will probably be more inclined to accept certification than many state rehabilitation counselors. It will help stabilize the job descriptions for many facilities and will again ensure the individual citizen or state agency that is purchasing the service from a facility or private counselor that a minimum level of competency has been established.

Third, for the state agency rehabilitation counselor the basic question will be whether the administration of the state accepts certification. It would appear at this time that there are a few state administrators highly in favor of certification and a few state administrators adamantly against certification. The biggest number of state administrators seem to be taking a middle of the road approach to certification and more or less a "wait and see" type of attitude. It would appear important that the individual rehabilitation counselor demonstrate through his own initiative that he has enough concern about certification that he move forward with certification regardless of where the state administrator stands on this issue. The state administrator will become more oriented toward certification if he sees his employees recognizing this as an important and beneficial asset. Most assuredly, unless the state administrator of a vocational rehabilitation program accepts and endorses certification, it will be a long, uphill task for the field of rehabilitation counseling to have certification standards as part of its basic philosophy. The state agency administrator will have to accept this as a meaningful direction in the field of rehabilitation before it will make a very dramatic impact on the field.

IMPACT AND IMPLICATIONS

It is difficult at this point in time to forecast the impact and implications that certification may have, but the following ideas come to mind in the discussion of certification and the ultimate impact and implications that it has for the field of rehabilitation counseling.

1. The *upgrading of services and professional recognition* is an implication that cannot be denied. Any time a profession sees within itself that it needs a minimum level of competency to assure client services then we automatically have an upgrading of services and a recognition of the profession by individuals outside of rehabilitation counseling based on that profession's own insight and concern to upgrade itself.

2. There will undoubtedly be an impact and implication for *education and training*. Inservice, regional training programs, and long-term training programs will have to attune themselves to the needs of the counselor who wishes to become certified. Certification is based on meeting certain criteria and by demonstrating competency in medical information, psycho-social aspects of

handicapping conditions, occupational information, and all the points previously covered. One of the very positive benefits that certification could give the educator or inservice training director is a sense of direction and purpose. It should be easier to plan specific conferences based on the areas of content determined to be necessary to move toward certification. This has the potential of unifying America's training effort in the field of rehabilitation counseling by focusing on the content areas described previously. This is particularly true for inservice training directors who will have the ability to conduct a program that will contribute toward the certification of the individual counselor. The counselor does not have to go through a long-term graduate training program to achieve the necessary academic competency areas, but rather this can be accomplished through state and staff inservice training.

3. *Counselor mobility.* In the years to come the implication for certification in counselor mobility becomes apparent. There are many counselors throughout the United States who are employed on a very political, or "who you know," basis. If state programs will adopt a policy of uniform employment standards based on the certification standards, then the mobility of the certified rehabilitation counselor will become easier. A counselor wishing to move from one part of the country to another will know whether or not he meets the standards of that particular job because they will be based on the background of certification.

4. *Professional bargaining power.* It would appear that one of the areas that could be strengthened is in the area of professional bargaining. Certification could create a solid front for political purposes as well as a definable legislative front for salaries. This would be the first time that on a nation-wide basis there would be similarity in backgrounds of all rehabilitation counselors based on meeting certain qualifications to become certified. This again throws us into the political arena, but in 1974 and the years henceforth this would seem to be where rehabilitation must focus much of its energy. To successfully do so, the rehabilitation counselor must be able to demonstrate that he has a base of competency above and beyond question.

5. *A sense of unity.* Throughout the United States there is a continuing morale question among rehabilitation counselors; not only "Who are we?" but more of a sense of "Are we somebody, and

are we being noticed?" Certification could have its impact in helping to unify the counselors in this country by making sure that each counselor had a clear-cut definition of his role and function and that his basic level of competency was shared by thousands of other counselors working in many other different states. One of the more difficult questions that rehabilitation is currently facing concerns the morale of people who are unhappy with their profession and seemingly are not quite sure what their profession is all about in the first place.

6. *State employment practice.* One of the major focuses that certification could have is in the change of civil service job descriptions. If certification is successful it will be measured by how well it can change job descriptions in every state in the nation. There will have to be a gradual state civil service change to reflect the certification movement.

7. *Private facilities.* Perhaps there will be a more immediate impact within private facilities. Private facilities have for some period of time had to undergo accreditation. State agency rehabilitation programs have often reviewed facilities in the determination of payment of fees. The earliest impact of certification will probably occur within private facilities wherein they will begin to change their job descriptions to reflect the certification standards. This will be a help to the total profession, and indeed it will help to demonstrate to rehabilitation as a whole the impact that certification is having.

8. *Accountability.* From almost any point of measurement, whether it be financial or client responsibility, accountability is a serious concern for the field of rehabilitation. Certification is just one step in meeting the accountability question, and it is a significant indication to the legislator and the disabled citizen alike that the profession is moving toward a professional thrust that heretofore has not been seen within rehabilitation.

These points and possibly many others hold implications for the future of rehabilitation based on the certification movement. These are only projections for the future, and any or all of them may have serious concern for the field of rehabilitation as we look at it in relationship to certification.

Stanley J. Smits

The Role and Function of the Rehabilitation
Counselor Serving the Severely Disabled

After defining and differentiating among counseling, rehabilitation counseling, and vocational rehabilitation counseling, the conclusion is reached that in working with the severely disabled, vocational rehabilitation counselors must broaden the scope of their services beyond that of "vocational" matters. For such clients, return to work is not equated with return to normalcy. Restructuring internal needs and long-term supportive counseling are both needed for the severely disabled. Provision of such services will require role changes for the rehabilitation counselor.

Heated arguments have permeated our field for almost twenty years regarding the ideal role and function of the rehabilitation counselor. In part, the basis for the debate has been a failure to differentiate among the numerous activities of a professional nature that are loosely referred to by the broad label of "counseling." Before attempting to discuss the issue of severe disability, I must first remove some of the confusion regarding traditional counseling services in State Rehabilitation Agencies. I will do so by presenting some of the differences I see among "counseling," "rehabilitation counseling," and "vocational rehabilitation counseling."

"Counseling" is a generic term in the area of human services. In its broad usage, it overlaps with "guidance" at one extreme and "psychotherapy" at the other. Guidance is a brief information exchange that attempts to direct a person toward appropriate decisions relevant to coping with his external environment. Psychotherapy, on the other hand, is a relatively long-term treatment process designed to reduce incapacitating emotional strife. It focuses on man's internal states. Counseling, as it was described in 1952 by those psychologists who were attempting to fill the gap between vocational guidance and psychotherapy, is a helping process during which a person is made more aware of his inner needs and explores alternatives for satisfying those needs within his environment. Counseling is especially important for psychologically normal people who find themselves in crisis from the death of a loved one, failure at work or school, marital stress, and so forth. It is also important for deviant populations who are attempting to approximate normal populations in activities of daily living. It is closely associated with developmental psychology.

As soon as we add the adjective "rehabilitation" to the noun "counseling," we give it new, more narrow parameters. It implies the existence of a disability and sets a goal of returning the client to normalcy. The adjective in this instance is capable of standing alone as a noun. When it does, "rehabilitation" denotes an array of services, counseling being one of them, designed to achieve a total rapproachment with disability. Rehabilitation counseling, then, is a helping process designed to assist in the total life adjustment to disability.

By adding "vocational" to "rehabilitation counseling," we give it a clear, specific target. The deviance from normalcy is the lack of a job; the lack of a job is in turn related to the existence of a disability. Vocational rehabilitation counseling focuses on removing and/or bypassing the obstacles to employment imposed by disability. It is much like "guidance" in that it is attempting to achieve success in an objective, predictable area in the person's environment. It is essentially an information exchange that matches the disabled client with a suitable job or with an educational or vocational treatment appropriate to developing his employment potential to the point of readiness.

Turning now to the concept of severe disability, it is my opinion that "rehabilitation counseling" as a broader treatment is needed rather than vocational rehabilitation counseling. I say this for several reasons. First of all, severe disability is a chronic problem that has substantial residuals after treatment is completed. Secondly, many life adjustment areas are involved. This means that a return to work is *not* equated with a return to normalcy. And finally, the ability to satisfy the severely disabled person's needs in his environment is so drastically reduced that a restructuring of his internal need hierarchy is needed in order to bring about concordance. This restructuring comes close to psychotherapy. However, counseling is an appropriate term for it because the person is attempting to resolve a crisis rather than deal with pathologic emotionality. Even after a restructuring of the need hierarchy has been achieved, long-term supportive counseling is needed to deal with the problems associated with chronicity.

If you accept my position, that vocational rehabilitation counselors must broaden the scope of their services well beyond "vocational" matters in order to serve the severely disabled, then you may want to consider the following role changes:

1. *Rehabilitation counselors will need to provide long-term services.* The service delivery system will need to change to accommodate (a) continuous services extended over many years, (b) a new method of measuring success other than a Status 26 Closure, and (c) a reward system to encourage counselors to persist with difficult cases.

2. *Rehabilitation counselors will need to work closely with family members.* Severe disability disrupts the entire family, not just one member. The successful containment of the debilitating effects of the disability requires the rehabilitation of the whole family.

3. *Rehabilitation counselors will need to become very familiar with homebound employment.* The severely disabled person has tremendous problems in the areas of transportation and self care. The development of homebound industries would bypass these problems and still allow productive activity.

4. *Rehabilitation counselors need to work more closely with other professionals.* We have talked the team approach to death in rehabilitation but actually used it only sparingly. The complex problems of the severely disabled make the team approach a necessity not a luxury.

5. *Rehabilitation counselors will need to become counselors.* For years we have provided a sophisticated "guidance" service to handicapped people whose feasibility for services meant something close to job-readiness. We merely guided them past the remaining obstacles and placed them in employment. With the severely disabled, we need to counsel, as I have used the term here, in order to help our clients deal with the psycho-social impact of a chronic, pervasive threat to their normalcy.

Program Implementation As It Relates to the Severely Impaired

Program implementation has not been optimally effective because of the rapid increase in the number of programs, clients, and staff. Particularly important for quality and quantity of client services are improved management techniques and the ability to delegate authority. In the light of recent congressional legislation, it becomes necessary to reexamine the role of the agency, renew commitments, rearrange priorities, and revise services. Two groups which will especially require expanded services are those of the more severely disabled and the deaf. Better utilization of the Governor's Committee can also result in improved program implementation.

I am amazed that there are so many people here. I rather expected to sit around a small conference with about a half dozen interested professionals and talk about what we needed to do to get under way toward our commitment to serve the severely disabled. When I walked into this room I was surprised to see such a tremendous gathering. It seems to me that all of us have had real growing pains, and this is part of our problem when we begin to talk in terms of what we should do in serving the severely disabled. I think we do have to make a strong and vigorous commitment to serving the physically and mentally handicapped. I think the statement that Congress doesn't expect a particular percentage of people to be rehabilitated was well put. Congress simply wants you to work with the handicapped.

You and I know that we digressed a long way away from working with physically and mentally handicapped when we began to include the so-called behavioral disorders. It began at the time when we started working with public offenders. We started blanketing almost everybody under the category of being disabled if they had two or three factors going for them. If they were intelligent and if they were disadvantaged, we could somehow or another find a handicap to go along with it. I can remember when we used to make high school surveys of the senior class at the end of the year, and the most eligible kid I ever found was one with an I.Q. of 120 and a modest handicap. That was the sort of client that we could send to college, and for four years we had our caseload up to a certain level without having to struggle with it. This boy would come back at the end of every quarter or semester and contact us. He'd make good grades, he'd go to work making $6,000 a year at the end of his graduation, he'd keep your average up, and this was the sort of client that we could find eligible very easily. I think that we've all had our share of the cases, and we continue to have our share of the cases relating to physical restoration. That's why I have had mixed feelings and sometimes have felt that it would be good to get rid of the physical restoration problem. I've also felt that there's a real need for physical restoration services to be provided by the rehabilitation program because of the importance of that service to the total rehabilitation of the client.

On the one hand I see in the future, the not too distant future perhaps, some medical care program that would be a nation-wide program to take care of a majority of our physical restoration problems. At the same time I see the importance of a continuation of an involvement with the client in order to make sure that your total product comes out inthe way that you'd have it come out. Now Jack Duncan, as you probably recognize, is a handicapped person. He wears a built-up shoe or perhaps shoes. He does have a decided limp. I believe that Jack was a client of the South Carolina agency. I remember Jack when he was on Mary Switzer's staff. I was very impressed with him then, and I was impressed with what he and Joe Owens had to say yesterday, and I hope you were. I took Jack and Joe and Craig Mills on a little tour of the City of Good Abode yesterday afternoon, and Jack made some comment about his disability. He didn't really elaborate, but apparently he has some difficulty with his old disability because he is going to have to have some medical attention. He said he was saving up his money, and Joe once told him, "Well, just put it off a couple more years and we'll find you a physician who's a GS-16, and it won't cost you much." This gives you an idea of the directions which people in Washington may be taking. They're really talking about an organized medical program. This almost sounds like the Harry Truman program of 1948 and socialized medicine. I don't know what Dr. Gardner's reaction to this would be, but I'm sure he'd agree that there are many forces at work, and we may arrive at some sort of guaranteed medical program sooner than we think. I can't predict when and don't even intend to; no one talks about this except to say that it is a part of the forces that affect us in our work. But I think we must have a serious commitment to working with the severely disabled if we're to continue as a viable program which serves people. Whenever you come so close to being abolished, as we were—well, we weren't really supposed to be abolished, but we were almost passed over as if we really didn't count or amount to a whole lot. There was an attempt made, as you well know, to abolish completely the OEO program. While the program wasn't completely eliminated, certain elements of it were dismantled.

If we have any real insight at all, we'll take this as the handwriting on the wall that says to us, "Look, you've got to make your program viable and you've got to meet the needs of today—it can't be a program that was typical in 1921 through 1939 and continue forever." It has to be the kind of program that meets today's needs. I think today's needs are geared to meeting the needs of the severely disabled. John Whitaker gave me an article not too long ago. One of the news magazines, probably *U.S. News and World Report*, indicated that the new minority group is the handicapped. This is a significant force in our social and governmental structure. The handicapped themselves have decided that they've got to get together; they've got to put pressure on the governmental agencies and the social agencies to get what they want and what they need. As an example, I think of the new underground subway that's being built in Washington, D.C., being built with no provisions for seriously handicapped persons getting in and out of the subway. As a result of this tremendous pressure, they now have to go back and put elevators at all the sites to the new subway, which is going to cost hundreds of thousands of dollars more than it would have cost had it been planned to accommodate the handicapped in the beginning. So we see on every hand where pressures are beginning to mount. The handicapped have taken lessons from some of the other minority groups, and they find that if they unite and demand services and exhibit a united front, they get action.

I think that too often we've talked of serving the severely handicapped but ended up serving the less severely handicapped. If our statistics are anywhere near accurate, there are plenty of seriously disabled people who need our service. We don't really have to expend our resources, time, and effort serving those who could probably serve themselves. While we're not calling a moratorium on serving the so-called three H's, I think that we see a trend toward finding other resources to serve clients who have hernias, hemmorrhoids, and hysterectomies that need to be performed. I hope we'll utilize those other resources to the extent that we can. I don't want anyone to be denied services. I think we found the same attitude on the part of the two people from Washington yesterday. Our commitment, they thought, was to serve more severely disabled persons more intensely and more successfully while at the same time continuing to serve the people we are now serving. Well, this is really a big order, so I think we really have to take a new look at things, and we have to adjust our method of operation.

We really can't serve the severely disabled if we just go back home and continue to do the same things we've done in the past. We have to have a new emphasis. We have to have a new push. We must focus the spotlight on a different approach. We're going to have to utilize the resources that are available. Some of you more or less represent facilities and institutions that have services to offer. Others represent the area of program management that needs services and are in a position to influence the purchase of service. We're going to need every resource, in my judgment, that we now have and can develop and utilize. We have twenty-one training centers across the state that are geared up (to a more or less degree) to provide a really fine evaluation and adjustment service. I don't think we've learned how to use them yet. We're still taking those clients with whom we don't know what to do, and we're sending them to the facility, hoping that some miracle will happen. I think we're nearing the time when we will look at a client on the basis of his needs and refer him to a facility for a particular service that will really help him to participate in the world of work. We're going to have to provide a kind of measured, planned program of services rather than just sending someone over to the training center hoping that some good will result. We've really not utilized our training centers as well as we should have. We've not given them the leadership that we ought to have given them. So we have got to get on with the show.

We have hundreds, well maybe not hundreds, but dozens, at least, of excellent private facilities. We've got Chet Scherman here this morning from Goodwill Industries in Knoxville. That program is turning out to be an excellent program, and their concern is our concern. If we have a need that is not being met, I find that the private agencies that manage facilities are anxious and eager to help us meet those needs. We simply have to identify our needs and bring them to their attention, and they're usually right there ready to try to help you solve the problem.

I think our commitment to the severely disabled is going to have to be strong; it's going to have to be a commitment that says we're really going to do something different; we're going to really emphasize this approach; we're going to do a job that we've not done in the past. I hope that we can also move ahead in a more vigorous way in employing the handicapped and in providing more opportunities of upward mobilization of our handicapped clients. I think we have talent on the staff that perhaps we're wasting—we've not really utilized certain abilities. I have difficulty expressing myself without making personal references, and I hope that in this group we can just "let our hair down" and talk about the things we need to talk about. For example, I think we're wasting Gene Taylor's talent. Gene Taylor probably has as good a mind as anybody we've got on the staff, and about the only thing we've let Gene do is to write evaluation reports after the other staff members have tested them. Now I'm not prepared at this point to say that we're wasting Gene's talents, but that's my impression. Maybe we ought to give Gene Taylor an opportunity to be a counselor. That's what he was trained to do. There are other opportunities, I think, that we overlook. We get in a rut. I hope that we'll take a new look at our own resources, those under our own command. We in the state office, and I guess this would be true of you regional directors, too often just get into a pattern of utilizing the same old resources, and we don't really look for new ways and improved ways of doing things.

This brings us to another area that I want to emphasize in terms of working with the severely disabled. It's always easier to tell the other guy what's wrong with his shop than it is to admit what's wrong with yours. I remember one time when we had a meeting over in South Carolina with rehabilitation people—public welfare folks and some personnel people. When we broke up into small groups to talk about the problems, I made the suggestion that what we ought to do is have the rehab folks get together and talk about what's wrong with welfare and let the welfare folks get together and talk about what's wrong with rehab. We can easily point out the deficiencies of that other department, but it's awfully hard for us to recognize our own. Therefore, I'm going to take the privilege of the chair, since I've got the microphone right now, and I'll let you have a chance later. I'm going to tell you what's wrong with the regional office, and later on you can tell us what's wrong with the central office. Is that a fair deal?

There are two or three points that I do want to make really seriously. I think each of us has to re-examine our role and the agency structure with respect to our commitment of serving the handicapped and, more particularly, our commitment to serving the *severely handicapped.* Now you know and I know that we just kind of grew up overnight in a way. This was not really a planned growth so much as it was a kind of explosive growth. Now when you grow so rapidly you may find all of a sudden that you're operating a big program with the same kind of management principles and tools that you used when you were a real small program. Doc Williams liked to refer to it as operating on a "personality basis." He'd say you can't do that, and I tend to agree with him. He says that we've outgrown the personality pattern of management and we ought to get into some scientific management principles and establish a program that we know will work. Well, maybe this is the theme of what I want to talk about. I think our regional directors have tried to maintain a big program in the same manner that they operated a small program; for example, the regional director has always been all things to all of his staff. I don't think we can do that any more. I don't think the regional director can spread himself thinly enough. There are not enough hours in the day for each regional director to respond directly and individually to each member of the staff with each problem that he has. I just don't think it's possible. I think the regional director has got to communicate with his staff through you, the supervisor. He's got to come to you with the problems that he sees as being management problems. He's got to turn them over to you and let you solve them. He's got to give you a commitment to go out and do a certain job for him, expect you to do it, and hold you accountable for it. I don't think there's any other way to do it.

They say confession is good for the soul, and I ought to feel good after this one, but that's one of my problems. I have a difficult time growing up to the point where I can assign the job to my staff and then make sure that they follow through and be held accountable for it. Well, you regional directors are going to have to do the thing that I'm not doing. I guess, and that is to understand what your major role is in relation to managing this program. Now please don't misunderstand me. I'm not suggesting for a minute that you ever give the impression to any member of your staff that you're not available to him at any time that he really needs you. That's one thing you've got to guard against very carefully. I think you've got to work hard to make sure your staff has the understanding that your door is open to them if they really have a problem. But what I am taking about is getting the job done through other people.

Now let's talk about you, the caseworker supervisor, for a moment. We'll talk as if the regional directors were not here, only we hope they'll listen. Too often you've ended up doing the sort of errand work or leg work that the regional director may not have time to handle because he hasn't relied on you from the outset. I don't think you ought to do this errand work for him. I realize you can't tell him to "go jump in the Mississippi River or the Tennessee River or Norris Lake"—that is if you want to stay around; but at the same time I think that you ought to be aware of your commitment, and he ought to be aware of the fact that you have a particular job to do, that you have twelve counselors under your supervision, and Lord knows that's too many. However, if you have eight counselors, twelve counselors, or whatever number, you've got a full time job in helping the counselor manage his caseload and provide services to people without having to do the regional director's job. That goes for our job too. We sometimes give you extra assignments. We call up and say, "Hey, how about doing so and so?" and, you know, you're always nice: you respond to it and you do just that for us instead of telling us to "go jump in the river" or get somebody else to do it.

I guess that what we're really saying is that we're going to have to put more time, more effort, more emphasis, and more planning on the casework process. We're going to have to work with counselors on the basis of working with the client. I think that the Program Appraisal Review ought to be done on a small number of cases to assist regional directors and provide some idea of the flavor of the situation in his region as compared to the rest of the state. I think that the major case reviews ought to be done by the casework supervisor. It ought to be done on a regular basis. You ought to be reviewing cases of the counselor under your supervision on a regular basis, not waiting until he's in trouble with a case. You ought to be working with the counselor on a planned basis by helping him to find the resources he needs to do the job for the severely disabled.

I guess what I am really saying is this: if you, as a casework supervisor, have a territory of two or three offices under your supervision, or one office and several counselors, you've got a full time job and a job that needs a lot of planning. You've got to plan and work with your staff on a regular basis. If you're going to see to it that the severely disabled get services, you're going to have to work with your counselors with that in mind. You're going to have to help them find the resources that they need to serve the severely disabled, and you're going to have to insist that counselors work with the severely disabled.

I've probably said more than I should have, but this is what we have to look at from time to time. I hope that some of you will tell us what we ought to do in the state offices; the Lord knows we need some help. There's no doubt in my mind that we sometimes spend more time spinning our wheels than we do getting to where we ought to be going. It's often a difficult task just to answer the phone and open the mail, much less get anything done, and that's getting to be a bigger job all the time. It seems to me that I work about half time for the telephone, and two-thirds time for the computer; the rest of the time my secretary is trying to get me to answer the mail. And I don't blame her. She should. I guess that each of us will have to grow up a little bit, and we may have to call on George Bass to help us develop some management techniques and help us find our way out of the woods. George is certainly willing to do that, and they've got some fine programs that are available.

We must attempt to focus on the kinds of things we need to do in order to make maximum use of our time. If we don't do that, we may be working eight, ten, eleven, or twelve hours a day, and now that we've got a commitment from the Department of Labor we can't do that. We're covered under the minimum wage, and you can't work your staff overtime. If you do you've got to pay them overtime; if you're not covered, you are entitled to compensatory time. There are all kinds of regulations you have to be aware of. We used to work around them. Now we've got hung up with them, just like Goodwill Industries has. I know you have your problems. I think if we're going to serve the severely disabled, we have to make a commitment to work with our staff on a planned and organized basis and on a regular basis. We're going to help them arrange the kind of medical consultations that they need. They're going to have their cases planned when they come. They're going to have an idea what they intend to do with them. They're going to have diagnostic services that suggest the sort of program you ought to plan for the client. If you don't provide these services they're going to send their clients to facilities where such services are available.

I want to make several other comments while I've got the floor, and then we're going to have some discussion. In our commitment to serve the severely disabled, I want us to include a special commitment to serve the deaf. I think we've got to serve the deaf to a greater degree than we have ever done. I know there is a tendency to say, "Well, you know, we're doing the best we can, and there really aren't very many deaf people out there, 'cause they don't come in for services, so I think we're doing about all there is to be done." But there are more deaf persons in this country than there are blind people, and yet we've got a staff of only a half a dozen people who are trying to work with the deaf, and we've got an entire program devoted to serving the blind with a staff of about seventy-five to one hundred people. I'm convinced that we would need to have as many people working for the deaf as Elaine Parker has on her staff working for the blind if we were really serving the needs of the deaf people.

If we don't move with some dispatch towards serving this group of people and doing it right away, I think we're going to have the kind of situation that occurred in Virginia. We'll have legislation to set up a commission of services for the deaf. Then we'll have three rehabilitation programs instead of two, and we'll be funding that just like we do with the program for the blind. I think it's high time we move vigorously ahead with serving the deaf. I want you to know what I've done. I brought Myra Luker to the state office. Ronnie was good enough to loan me the person and the position. Jerry made a commitment before he became regional director. I forgot to ask him after he got to be regional director if he'd do that, but, anyway, we have brought Myra to the state office, simply a position move, and we've asked Myra to head up a program of serving the deaf. Now

Jerry did a fine job of that when he was in our state office. I think Jerry would admit himself that he does not have the expertise or the skill or the knowledge to work directly with deaf persons and communicate with deaf person, and it seems to me that Jerry and I and the rest of you are at a distinct disadvantage if we can't communicate with the deaf; you don't really get much conversation going. I guess that's one way of saying the same thing twice, isn't it? At any rate, unless you can sign or communicate with the deaf in some way, you don't really get much of a relationship going.

The model state plan that has been developed and submitted by a task force of NRA (which was discussed in the Tucson Conference on serving the deaf) is a model for states that have done very little in terms of serving the deaf and a guideline to other states to try to do a better job. We want to implement in this state, I think, the model state plan. Myra is going to be our central office coordinator in serving the deaf, and she'll be around to talk with you as time goes on, particularly the regional directors and the staff in your region that work with deaf persons. We were fortunate enough to get Craig Mills to have breakfast with us this morning and to share some ideas they are using in the state of Florida.

Now I make this statement; I think it's a fair statement to make (I base it purely on my own particular make-up and how difficult it was for me to finally understand that there is a real problem in working with deaf persons, and there is a big job to be done). I think those staff members who are working with the deaf have to be extremely cautious that they don't give the impression to the deaf that they really aren't sincere or they they really aren't committed. I think you have to work very carefully with deaf persons. They seem to be rather sensitive in terms of the way they perceive things, and then, too, there is such a communication gap that sometimes they don't hear what you say; they hear what they think you said, and this can be very different. I think we also have to work carefully with those who are not committed to working with the deaf and try to convince them that there is a problem. These staff members have the particularly difficult task of convincing both you and the deaf community that they are really sincere in working. I guess they may have a double-barrelled handicap. I believe that we should give them our support. We should vigorously support expansion of services to deaf persons, and there really are more deaf persons than we have ever imagined. They don't seek our services because they don't feel that they get adequate services. We've made some surveys and that is exactly what the surveys say. They don't think there is any point in coming to rehab because rehab has never done anything for them. So I think we've got to change that image and this is as good a time as any to do so because deaf persons are certainly classified as severely disabled; this is a good way to increase our commitment to the severely disabled.

There are one or two other things on which I might comment. I think our Governor's Committee is a force that we've not really utilized. We've kind of tolerated it. That's not a very good thing to say, I guess, but in a way this is what we've done. There is no reason why the Governor's Committee ought not to be a tremendously powerful, dynamic force in working with the severely handicapped person. They've got all sorts of opportunities to open up avenues for us and our counselling staff that we just overlook time and again. There has been a problem of communication, I think, within our state office and within our regional offices about just what the Governor's Committee is supposed to do and the nature of its assignment. Now if there is any misunderstanding, let me take the major responsibility for that right now, and I'll tell you why it's that way, and then maybe we can devise a way to keep it from being that way.

When we first started to fund some positions for the Governor's Committee, it seemed to us that it was extremely important that we keep every other agency, both state and federal, involved to the extent possible with the employment of the handicapped. So we bent over backwards, I think, to make certain that everybody understood that the Governor's Committee belonged to all of the public agencies, that it represented Welfare, Employment Security, the U.S. Department of Labor, and the Veterans Administration to the same degree that it does the Division of Vocational Rehabilitation. I think everybody knows now that we're funding the Governor's Committee, and we finally admitted that they are part of our unit, and we just moved them in with us in the state office. There is no real reason for us to present a front that says, "You know this is a separate function." Now it is separate and I think it's recognized as separate, and I want it always to be a program that can cut across all lines. There is a very distinct need to have the kind of communication with other agencies that the Governor's Committee can make possible.

I think we can improve on that, but I also think we've missed the boat in not being a greater part of helping the Governor's Committee plan a program that meets the needs of our clients. So I want us to correct that. I want you directors and supervisors and central office staff to give thought and attention to the kind of program you think the Governor's Committee ought to provide for the handicapped people in this state. Now I don't believe any of you think that they ought to be a placement agency. Of course, if you do think so, let's have that recommendation, because we ought to deal with that kind of possibility if it's viable.

I do believe there is a very vital role that they can serve for the severely handicapped person in the state, and I think we need all the forces we can get working in that direction. I see a role that is emerging; I hope you are aware of it, and I hope that it will be a viable and beneficial role for you. I think the Governor's Committee can play a distinct, vital role in working with industry and not only open up opportunities for handicapped persons to be employed, but also perhaps provide training for people in industry in how to work with handicapped persons. Charlie Lenox called to my attention a program that the TVA is trying to put into effect in their own shop, and he was kind enough to get the package for me from Ed Hilton which they acquired from the state of Texas. Texas has developed an entire program, training industry supervisors to work with handicapped people. It's about a six- or seven-hour course, and it's developed on a behavior modification approach. You take it directly into the plant. You spend one day with your plant supervisor, and give them a pretest. You provide this training during the next six hours, and it's amazing how much of a change of attitude you can achieve in one day. The success of the handicapped persons on the job means that the employer will come back to you for additional handicapped persons to be employed in that industry. I don't see how we could provide a greater activity for the severely handicapped than to assure their success on the job once they get a job. So this is an area to which the Governor's Committee might very well give some consideration.

The Governor's Committee is in the process of making a survey of industry in determining that attitude of industry toward serving handicapped persons. Now you and I know that as the jobs become more scarce, the more severely handicapped person is usually the first to go and the last to be hired, which means we're going to have a doubly difficult job to do. We're going to serve the severely disabled at a time when the economy is in a decline. So again, I think we need all the forces we can muster to do the job. Our Workmen's Compensation cases need additional attention, and we're now working on that. I think Bob is working with Miss Johnson to try to bring about a new contract. I don't know what's happening to Jerry with BEC. I believe Spivey came up to see us some months back, but we haven't had any contact with him lately. I don't know what our experience has been with respect to getting plans approved for BEC to pay what the services cost. This is something we need to look into, but I think that we're going to have to work more vigorously with Workmen's Compensation cases and the industrial accident cases for two reasons. One is to assist those person to regain employment and to assist those who haven't worked to become employed.

Ed Hilton and Jane Harrison, who have been counselors with this staff for a long time, are now both working with TVA. They've come to the conference for the VSRA meeting, and I invited them to come early for this meeting. They tell me that TVA's compensation load alone is $7 million a year for persons who have been disabled on TVA jobs. And the projection is that by 1985 this will be $21 million unless something drastic is done to correct this. So you can see that there is a substantial problem, not only in TVA but other industry as well, in terms of the compensation load for disability. TVA has embarked on a positive action program to employ the handicapped, but first of all and, perhaps more importantly, to concentrate on trying to re-employ those persons who've been disabled in TVA accidents. This may give you a little idea of the size of the problem that you encounter with the severely disabled and with the Workmen's Compensation cases. Lord knows how many we have, but there are plenty to work with. In working with the severely disabled there are two good resources that we can look toward in getting the kinds of cases that we need to really be working with.

There is one other area that we need to continue to give attention to, or give more attention to, perhaps, than we have in the past. We're going to be in a period of consumer participation for some time. I don't know how long. It's going to be difficult to project how long this will continue, but I think we're right in the midst of a time when the consumer will have a strong voice in suggesting what is delivered to him, both at the retail counter level or the government service level. It's going to become more complex before it gets simpler. We've got to be concerned about how the consumer feels about the product that we're trying to deliver to him. We've got to get more in tune with what our clients feel they need and desire. We have to constantly be alert to working with communities, community groups, with individuals, so that we can come up with the kinds of things that will help us to remain a viable, dynamic program that can shift with the times and meet the needs of today and plan for the needs of tomorrow.

William M. Williams

Guideline Interpretation

Of primary importance to the implementation of the 1973 Rehabilitation act is the identification of those "severely disabled" to whom the act gives first priority of services. Identifying characteristics of the severely disabled, as opposed to those of non-severely disabled, are reported. It is suggested that evaluation of the functional limitations of these groups be carried out through vocational training centers and through private, non-profit making centers. Evaluation is seen as the key to successful provision of services.

There's been a lot said about serving the severely disabled, not only at this conference, but also for the last several years. Now with the advent of the 1973 Rehabilitation Act it has become law. We have tried to keep the regional directors on board because they along with the staff will have to implement the mandate. In visualizing and realizing what lies ahead, we've tried to take into account the importance of identifying the severely handicapped because we feel that this is an area we are lacking in. However, I've not really heard anyone identifying the severely disabled. We have been provided codes and instructions to identify this group, but the grey area is broad and subjective.

Now if I'm correct, the national average is about 32 per cent severely disabled of all rehabilitation closures. The Tennessee percentage is about 27. I think here again we're dealing with an identification problem. I think it suggests to the counselor that he needs the help of the supervisors. You heard Ed Reece say that the supervisors have certain supervisory functions to perform. The counselor, too, has certain functions to perform, and I hope sincerely that we can provide some help for both the supervisor and the counselor and concentrate on the client and less on the paperwork process. I use this as an illustration because I was in St. Petersburg about three weeks ago along with Sid Corban and Bobby Brooks, and we were shown a proposed new format for a Plan of Services. There were seven pages involved, which to us represents entirely too much paperwork. At

77

any rate, Tennessee at the end of the fiscal year 1973-74 rehabilitated 27 per cent severely disabled people, which I consider low. I think if we had a more sophisticated identification process that the true figure would be somewhere closer to 35 to 40 percent. I would hope that we would shoot for this percentage. I think that once we start to really identify these cases, the percentage will increase.

The severely disabled person, by federal definition, is one who has a severe disability where a physical or mental impairment seriously limits the functional capacities, that is, the mobility, communication, self-care, self-direction, and work tolerance, to the extent that the person is unable to a substantial degree to cope with the physical or mental means of gainful employment and whose rehabilitation normally requires multiple services both restorative and compensatory, along with selective placement, over an extended period of time. Now they don't tell us what the extended period of time is. They have never told us what the extended period of time is, and this is what we're reckoning with. This is part of the identification process problem. How do you define an extended period of time? If what we're going to have to do is reckon with this, whether it's one year, two years, or three years, then hopefully in the guidelines we will eventually be given instructions so that we can deal with the problem down at the grassroots level. Hopefully, the supervisor will get involved and "guide" the counselor as to what an extended period of time is. Now it is up to us as supervisors, regional directors, and counselors to work together to identify the severely disabled. When we start to identify cases as being public assistance related or being severely disabled, based on a definition which we understand, then we will move out. But I think it behooves us not only to want to identify them but also to serve them. That's what we're faced with, and we're going to have to do that.

Further, I think it behooves us as supervisors to get with the counselors and help them work with severely disabled. It might be helpful to identify some of the characteristics of the severely disabled vs the non-severely disabled client:

Sex: There are more males in the severely disabled group: 71 per cent compared to 66 per cent.

Race: There are fewer *minorities* in the severely disabled group: 5 per cent are non-white compared to 12 per cent non-white in the non-severely disabled group.

Age: The severely disabled group is older than the non-severely disabled group; that is, 66 per cent of the severely disabled group are above the age of forty compared to the 33 per cent of the non-severely disabled group.

Education: The severely disabled group is less well educated (30 percent have an eighth grade or less education compared with 20 per cent in the non-severely disabled group).

Martial Status: The severely disabled group has more married persons (49 per cent are married compared to 29 per cent in the non-severely disabled group).

Number of Dependents: The severely disabled group has larger families (77 per cent have two or more family members compared to 65 per cent of the non-severely disabled).

Source of Support: Fewer of the severely disabled group are supported through personal sources or public assistance (only 12 per cent of the severely disabled group are receiving public assistance compared to 18 per cent of the non-severely disabled).

Monthly Income: Severely disabled have a higher monthly income at acceptance than the non-severely disabled group ($325 compared to $205 for the non-severely disabled).

Source of Referral: Most of the severely disabled group is referred by Social Security with very few coming from corrections, mental hospitals, and schools. Eight per cent of the severely disabled group were referred from the latter three sources compared with 34 per cent of the non-severely disabled. (The above information was printed in *Consumer Brief*, Vol. 2, No. 3, May, 1974).

The situation is this. Referrals are coming from Social Security, and I'll venture to say that within a few months they are going to be coming from SSI just like they're coming from SSDI. We're going to be receiving statutory—you call them what you want—legislative, and regulative referrals. I'll venture to say that the money is going to come from RSA with the rehabilitation of the SSI and SSDI client. That's what it's all about.

I want to summarize what the implications are for the counselors because you as a supervisor need to be involved with the counselor in identifying the severely disabled. The Rehabilitation Act of 1973 states that the priority will be on the serving of the severely disabled and then the "other" handicapped. I think that both groups can best be identified through the network of (1) vocational training centers and (2) the private, non-profit-making evaluation centers such as Goodwill and the institute of Human Resources. I think that these evaluation facilities can determine to what extent a client has functional limitations. For instance, can the client (1) climb one flight of stairs or walk one hundred yards; (2) lift fifty or one hundred pounds; and (3) coordinate sufficiently to be able to button buttons, wind a watch, or write with a pen? If evaluation is not a major function of the training centers then I don't know what the function of the training centers is ever going to be. I think that our training centers represent a great resource, I think we have the evaluation facilities to work with the severely disabled and to help us identify them. I think that once we realize this we'll become professionals. I have said over and over that if we're over going to become professionals then we're going to have to evaluate. No longer can we flip a coin, and if it comes up heads we send the person to beauty school, if it comes up tails we send her to business school. Once we start to really evaluate work we can help the severely disabled, and I think that therein lies the secret in evaluation.

I'm open for questions, and I'd appreciate some answers as far as the Rehabilitation Act of 1973 is concerned.

Data Processing

Although planning toward computerization of the total client services program began in 1967, lack of funds for equipment and accounting staff, plus the rapid increase in client services, caused many problems and delays.

In 1972, the state established a central computer complex, the Information Systems Service Division, which would incorporate the computer systems from all departments. A new data-processing system was designed to provide for the needs of Vocational Rehabilitation. Implementation of the new system was scheduled for July 1, 1975, but technical problems and insufficient key-punch staff for the workload caused delays in full use of the program.

Advantages in time-saving and in convenience will result when the program is fully operative, both for state and field offices. Emphasis must be placed on the necessity of providing timely and accurate information to the computer.

There's a slight correction on your program. If you'll notice, the topic is listed as Date Processing, so there just needs to be a slight change in the topic. Unfortunately, my involvement happens to be more with the corrected topic rather than with the one that is printed.

In June, 1967, I believe it was, representatives from the Department of Education's Data Processing Section and the Division of Vocational Rehabilitation went to Charlottesville, Virginia, to attend an Automated Systems Workshop. After returning from this meeting, they were thoroughly convinced that this was the way that we should go, to computerize our total client services program. Shortly after this meeting we began working with the systems and programming people from the Department of Education's Data Procession Section. The goal was established that the program would be complete and ready for implementation on July 1, 1968.

We proceeded on this basis and worked towards this goal; much effort was put into this program. We had numerous problems with it and finally reached the point where we had to make the decision whether to go or not go on. To solve these problems would require additional money and additional time, and unfortunately we were out of both at that particular time, so that program had to be scratched. We had to return to our old data processing system that we had been using. This is not completely correct, as far as returning to our old system, because in the time that the new program had been in the design stage and also the attempted implementation, our program had grown so much and our volume of work had increased so much that we could not continue to do the same things that we had been doing under our old system, so we had to scratch some of the things we were doing in order to accommodate our antiquated accounting machine. Prior to this time we had been punching up the information on each case as the different sections (R-300) came into the central office. We could take these cards and sort them and get some data about what our caseloads consisted of or information that we needed for management purposes. This is one of the things we had to discontinue in order to keep the bill paying process going.

For a period of time after this venture, we attempted to secure approval for the division to acquire a small computer in order to carry out our bill paying or financial transactions in a faster method. This approval was never secured so we had to continue plugging along like we had been doing. We had anticipated using the small computer in the bill paying process with the hope that at a later date it could be used as a terminal into a larger computer complex.

In the spring of 1972 the (then) Commissioner of Finance Administration had resigned. It was in the latter stages of the session of the legislature when this took place, or at least became known. The incoming commisioner was on the scene and was in the process of looking into the problems of the state to see what he was about to get into. One of the things that came to his attention was a complaint from a vendor or some vendors about the length of time it was taking to get their money from Vocational Rehabilitation. The Commissioner paid us a visit to look into our program and see what our problem was and what it would take to solve this situation. He assigned some of his staff from the Management Services Division to come out and do a study of our program to see what changes could be made. The result of this survey indicated the same thing that we had been trying to call to the attention of officials up the line for a couple of years—that we needed additional staff in our accounting section and that we needed an up-to-date data processing system. Along about this same time there was also a statewide study being conducted by an outside consulting firm to determine what the state's needs were for data processing. The combination of these two studies, the one by F.A., and also the consulting firm, resulted in a high priority being given to Vocational Rehabilitation for getting some kind of a new data processing system under way.

In 1972, the Governor issued Executive Order No. 18 that took all of the computer systems from the various departments and put them into a central computer complex known as Information Systems Services Division, or ISSD as it's more commonly called. A team of the staff in the Systems Development Unit was assigned to Vocational Rehabilitation to start designing our new system to take care of our needs. One area where we had problems with our earlier attempt to use the Department of Education's system was that there were a number of personnel changes in the analyst and the programming staff over the period of time that we were working with them. Also, their equipment really didn't have the capacity to handle our program. In working with the ISSD people we have worked with the same key staff for the past two years, which has certainly been to great advantage. With the central computer complex they should have the capacity to handle our program.

Insofar as vocational rehabilitation is concerned, we may appear to them to be a small organization, but they don't realize that in looking at our unit, compared dollar-wise to some of the other larger departments, we process a heck of a lot more paper to spend our few dollars than some of these other departments, because we're nickel and diming it to death, where everybody else is spending theirs in hundreds of thousands and millions of dollars lump sums. So the volume of paperwork that it takes to process our program is considerable.

It's difficult to list in any kind of order or priority or sequence the things that the new system is supposed to do because each one of them is so important. Those of you who have been in our central office in the accounting section have seen the numerous kardex filing cabinets that house the individual cost cards of active clients who have had an authorization issued for them. The hand posting operation has been taking place for a number of years. As each authorization comes into the central office it has to be audited and posted to this cost card. The same thing occurs when the bill comes in. It has to be audited and then posted on this cost card against an authorization. The new system is designed to eliminate this hand posting operation.

Under the new system, a client file is to be established. All the information that we gather on a client will be fed into this file at various times. This also applies to authorizations and payments. They will also go in this client file where they will become part of the total client file. The client file will give us management information we have not had for a long period of time. When we had to go back to our old data processing system, we had to give up keeping our file that we had at the time on clients. Since then the only information we have had in punchcard form has been on the cases that have been closed. We have been able to sort these whenever time was available on our equipment to get the information that we needed from closed cases. However, this never gives us information on our current caseload—the actual cases that we are working with—or problems we are having in caseload management. The new client file should give us the capability of getting this information. Quite often we need to know how many cases we are serving of a certain type of disability or we need some other management information, and we just don't have the capability of getting it through the central office records. The only way we can get it is to go back to the field and ask the counselor or the secretary to survey the caseloads and get this information for us and send it in to us. Quite often it is too time consuming to go this route and we just have to do without it. At other times it has been necessary to do this when we have had to have it. The new client file, when it is established, will give us the ability to get this information in the central office.

When the case is ready to close and all the R-300 information has to be sent to Washington, this will come off the client file. It will be sent to Washington in the form of a computer tape rather than on punch cards as we do now. This will eliminate the necessity of completing the R-300 at the time the case is closed because this information will be coming into the client file as the case progresses. At the same time as the case is closed, a document will be printed out which will be called the client profile. It will be a summary of all the information on that case for the life of the case. It will be sent back to the district and this client profile can be put in the folder and serve as a summary of the case.

Various monthly and quarterly statistical reports are now being prepared by the local offices, but we will be able to prepare these from the client file, so this is one process that will be eliminated. The master list prepared from the client file will be sent out to the districts on a monthly basis. At the same time an exception list will be prepared. It will show cases that have been in certain status for excessive periods, and this will enable us to have better caseload management. All the reports that will have to be housed in this file will require that the information going into the file be timely and accurate. Just as the changing of one letter in the topic of this discussion completely changed the topic, so will one incorrect digit in a client number completely foul up the client record. These records on the client file will be on there by client number order. The name of the client won't mean anything so far as actually calling up the information on file because the computer will have to look up this information by the client number and district number. An incorrect number could actually put information for a particular client in the wrong client's file.

Contrary to what some people think, a computer can't think, at least the present day computers can't. A computer is only a machine that can do things at a fantastic rate of speed. I cut out a little statement some years ago; it's been so long ago I don't even remember what I cut it out of, and I taped it on to one of the file boxes on my desk. It says, "Thinking optimistically, it would take fifty people working day and night for 200 years to make the same mistakes that an electronic computer could make in only two seconds." This is a kind of backhanded way of saying how fast the computer can work. But the mistakes that you hear of so often that the computer makes are not really the mistakes of the computer. It's the mistake of the input data that we put into the computer or the programming errors that were made to begin with, so it gets back to the data and the people involved and not just the computer itself. And again I say, the new system will require timely and accurate information. For example, the system will not accept an authorization on a client unless the client is in the proper status. This is something that we have not had the ability to audit in the past in the accounting section.

The question now is "Where are we on implementing this new system?" and that's a good question. It was scheduled to get into operation on July 1, but it didn't. In building the new client file this meant that all the data on the clients were out in the field, in the district, and in counselors' offices. We had none of it in the central office as we used to. We had to go back to the field and ask that all this information be sent into us. We realized at that time that we did not have the capability of punching all of this information into cards in order to feed these cards into the computers. We secured a contract with a private concern to do this additional keypunch work. During the early stages we had good turn around on this contract. We got the bulk of this work done with reasonable turn around. During the past few months, with the additional work that we have needed to have done, they have not given us satisfactory turn around and this has created some problems. Our keypunch staff consists of six people, three punchers and three verifiers. During the month of June, when our workload is extremely heavy (we always have an unusually large number of bills to pay during the month of June), we had only about 75 per cent of our keypunch time available because of absences of our staff. One of our operators was out for an extended period of time due to injuries received in an automobile accident. In anticipation of the additional workload, we budgeted for two additional keypunch operators. We submitted the necessary papers to get these positions established in time to get them filled by July 1. There was an unusually long delay in getting these papers approved. We were not able to fill these positions until some time in the latter part of July. So here again we had a lack of keypunch time. We have, because of these additional delays, requested that our keypunch staff be permitted to work overtime. This request was submitted back in July. Being optimistic, we thought that we would get approval within a couple of weeks. The request was for working through September 30 on overtime. When I left the office Monday we still had not heard from this request. Where we were hoping to get a two-months' period of overtime work, now one month is already going without securing any approval on this, so we're still not able to cut into this backlog of work that we have.

Our payments are currently being processed on the computer rather than on our old accounting machine that we had. These payments are being processed around the system and not through the system as it was designed. In doing this, we have had to continue the hand posting operation in the accounting section in order to do the necessary auditing and editing of these as they go through, since we cannot depend on the computer at this time or at least the system as it was designed. In trying to get the new system going or the new payment system, there have been problems simply because it's new. We secured a terminal that is located in our office out on West End that feeds into the computer that is located up town. In trying to take care of this payment process, there have been some problems in feeding the information into this terminal and getting it into the computer and getting the work back to us.

There have also been some other problems. The Division of Accounts has been designing a new accounting system known as the Financial Information Control System, better known as FICS. The new FICS system involves the use of vendor file, and Vocational Rehabilitation is being used as one of the guinea pigs in getting the new system going. It has been our vendors who have been used to create the file. I'm not certain, but I think that the Purchasing Division may also be on this at the same time, or at least Purchasing and Vocational Rehabilitation are the two that were going to be the prime users or the guinea pigs to do the testing. So we've had the combination of insufficient keypunch time, a new system going on the computer, which always presents problems, and then the new system in the Division of Accounts, which also presents problems. It has been pretty hectic trying to keep things going under all these conditions.

The vendor file that is being set up in the Division of Accounts under its system also is going to have to have accurate information. Each vendor is going to be identified by a vendor number and a location code, so each statement of account as it comes into the central office has to have these two identification numbers on it. The expenditure card that we punch up has this information punched into it as it is fed into the computer. The computer takes this number, looks it up on the vendor file and prints the check to the name of the individual or company that is on the file for this number. If the bill comes into the central office with the incorrect number, or if an inncorrect number is punched into the card, then the check is written to the wrong person. There is another visual audit that will have to be done to catch these. It is extremely important that this information be accurate when it comes into the central office. If a vendor moves, this information needs to be corrected on the file. The purpose of having this location code is to take care of one vendor who might have several offices in a particular location and payments going to several different places. Keep in mind that when we make payments to a client (for maintenance) the client is a vendor, so if that client moves the vendor file must be updated to show his new address or his maintenance payment will be mailed to his old address.

As it stands now, we are making our payments around the system by use of the computer, and we've had some problems with that. We think these problems should clear up fairly soon. The Division of Accounts and its problems with the vendor file will improve. Part of the problem with the vendor file is also keypunch time. As hard pressed as we have been for keypunch time, Carl Corlew volunteered to take some work of the Division of Accounts and keypunch it for them in order to update the vendor file so we could get our payments through.

Our major problem is the lack of our own keypunch time. The longer that we go without getting the additional keypunch time, the more problems this is going to create in getting the system implemented, because we have to go back to July 1 to bring the system up to date if it's going to be meaningful for the full year. I understand the frustrations that the field offices probably have been going through concerning payments to the vendor because we are going through the same frustration in the central office. I want to thank you for your cooperation in this venture and ask for your continued understanding and help in trying to get the system operational.

Discussion of Chapter 839 of Public Acts (1972) Relating to Providing Services to the Severely Impaired

Provisions of the Tennessee act providing for mandatory education of the handicapped are discussed. Outstanding features of this legislation include the concept of the least restrictive alternative, inclusion of the handicapped in the vocational education and placement program, and due process and rights of children provisions. Specific requirements of the act are examined with regard to implementing, funding, and changing current procedures and programs.

During the 87th General Assembly, in the closing minutes a bill that has been looked upon by educators throughout the state of Tennessee both as a blessing and as a curse was introduced and passed. For the handicapped child and for the parents of handicapped children, this bill, which we are now calling Mandatory Education of the Handicapped, represents a "Bill of Rights" for the education of handicapped children. It has been referred to as "Chapter 839." The educational of handicapped children became mandatory with the signing of this bill by Governor Dunn two years ago. The specific requirements of the Act include, but are not limited to, the following:

1. Local school systems are to provide special educational services sufficient to meet the needs and maximize the capabilities of handicapped children, ages four through twenty-one, by the fall of 1974. The bill provides that each local school system in the state assume the responsibility for handicapped children who reside in that school district. We have 146 school district in the state, so in effect we have 146 local education agencies that are charged with the responsibility of seeing that the handicapped who reside in their area receive quality special education instruction.

2. To the maximum extent practical, handicapped children shall be educated along with children who do not have handicaps and shall attend regular classes. This is probably causing a little bit of a problem as far as the cooperative program is concerned. I have hopes that we can really tackle this within the next two or three weeks and come up with some answers as to what the future will be of the work study program.

3. All school buildings shall be designed, constructed, and equipped to accommodate the requirements of any handicapped child likely to be served therein. This is a "bigee." It's a real "bigee." Right now we have a $300 million comprehensive vocational program that is getting off the ground which is designed to build comprehensive vocational schools which any boy or girl in the state of Tennessee will have an opportunity to attend. All of these schools will meet this specific criteria. As they are being planned, they must be planned for utilization by handicapped children.

4. It is the responsibility of local governments and local school systems to expend effort on behalf of each handicapped child equal to the effort expended on behalf on the non-handicapped child. Any additional effort necessary to provide supplementary aids and services shall be the responsibility of the state. What does this mean? It means that from this point on, local school systems must provide for the handicapped child not less than what they are spending on the non-handicapped child.

5. The bill provides that the State Commissioner of Education shall develop a comprehensive plan for implementing the policy set forth in the Act which includes (1) a census of all handicapped children in the State of Tennessee; (2) provisions for diagnostic and screening services for handicapped children; (3) an inventory of personnel and facilities; and (4) an analysis of the respective responsibility of various units of state and local government for providing special education services. This analysis is just beginning. We're starting next week to work in depth with the Department of Mental Health, Department of Public Health, Department of Correction, and other units of government, such as the State Planning Office, in trying to delineate areas of responsibility. We shall produce standards for the education to be received; produce a program for the preparation and recruitment of personnel; a program for the development, acquisition, con-

struction, and maintenance of facilities to implement the Act; and any other matters including recommendations for legislative change.

The bill also provides for the establishment of materials and training units to assist in the education of handicapped people and the establishment of parent review procedures for pupil placement. This is a strong section of the bill. The bill's action made due process a part of the school structure for the first time in the history of education in the state of Tennessee. We have specific wording in the legislation that says the parents of children and children themselves have certain rights and that these rights must be respected. Policies of the act also include the establishment of a plan to provide financial aid to school districts.

During this last year, we started planning for the implementation of the Mandatory Education of the Handicapped Act, and several tasks were completed during the last school year. First, we conducted a census throughout the state of Tennessee. Each school district was asked to conduct a complete census of all children who had been identified and verified as handicapped children and then to make some estimate about the number of additional youngsters who resided in the school district who probably were handicapped. Second, we completed a plan for local school system participation in the 1973-74 initial implementation of the Act. This provided for screening and diagnostic services, supervisory services, training of personnel, inservice education of personnel, and special projects. During the last school year, we funded this portion of the Special Education Program with $5.5 million that was allocated by the legislature for planning purposes.

During the year, we completed policies governing the development of programs and services for the handicapped. These policies were presented to the State Board of Education on April 5, 1974, and were approved. We completed a revision of the Rules, Regulations, and Minimum Standards. This was approved at the same board meeting in April. These regulations include the stipulation that local school systems should serve all verified handicapped children ages four through twenty-one during this school year, with the exception of the deaf. The legislation specifically allows us to go down to three years of age in education of the deaf, and, through an administrative decree by the Commissioner, in serving the deaf child or the hearing impaired child we are allowed to go to age zero or to birth. The rules and regulations also gave redefinition of evaluation and assessment procedures to be used in the unification and provided for the adoption of the distribution formula that reimburses a school system on the basis of how services are rendered. This distribution formula is possibly the most unique thing that we've done during the past year. It probably will be a forerunner for changing the whole distribution process to the schools in the state of Tennessee. Provisions of the Act also defined program service alternatives which recognize the concept of the least restrictive alternative, which means placement of pupils nearest to the regular classroom program as possible.

The following is a comparison of handicapped pupils served and the state appropriation for the handicapped for a three-year period. In the year 1972-73, or two school years back, we served by head count 60,347 youngsters in the state of Tennessee. For that school year, $16 million was appropriated by the legislature. Last year in the 1973-74 term, we actually served some 10,000 more, or an approximate total of 70,000 youngsters. Last year our total appropriation from state funds for the education of the handicapped amounted to $26 million. For the current 1974-75 school year, we originally projected that we would try to serve 85,000 pupils because 85,000 youngsters had been identified and verified as handicapped children. We had an appropriation by the legislature this year in the amount of $38,500,000. In planning for this 1974-75 school year, funds in the amount of $4,750,000 have been set aside for indirect services to handicapped children. The remaining state appropriation in the amount of $33,750,000 was budgeted for direct services for 85,000 children. Local school systems were asked to develop plans and submit them to the state by July 1, 1974, and advise us how they were going to serve the handicapped children who resided in their school districts. Instead of 85,000 pupils showing up on these plans that were developed and presented to the state by 146 school systems, 100,000 pupils were identified throughout the state of Tennessee. You don't have to be too proficient in arithmetic to know that this has resulted in some real problems. In fact, these plans that were submitted on July 1 of this year reflected requests for money in the amount of 146 per cent of the amount appropriated. We exceeded all our wildest expectations in trying to "get this problem off the ground."

We probably succeeded too well in developing this program at the beginning. Budget requests at 146 per cent amounted to something like $40 to $50 million, rather than the $38.5 million allocated by the state.

In order to stretch our funds to the maximum the use of federal funds from various discretionary programs, which may be used for programs for the handicapped, is planned for the state level services. For example, three instructional materials and training units—one in Jackson, one in Smyrna and one in Knoxville—are planned by the Division of Field Services and Resources. We expect to spend between $800,000 and $1 million during this school year in setting up these instructional materials centers. We're getting the funds for establishing these centers from ESEA Title II Funds in the amount of $225,000. The remaining money is derived from Education of Handicapped Act, Title VI Funds. These centers will employ approximately thirty-five to forty people and will provide technical and consultant services, materials and equipment to all school systems in the state. The magnitude, the bigness of this, is overwhelming, really. Three instructional material centers in the state of Tennessee will not do the job. We know it. Therefore, we will have satellite centers developed by local school systems or the cooperative systems that are currently developing in the state. Every effort will be made to coordinate ESEA Title I local grants. Vocational Education has set aside money which could be combined with any new federal appropriations and available state funds in order to serve the verified population of 100,000 during this year.

When we identified 100,000 individuals instead of 85,000, we had no choice but to attempt to serve these children. Therefore, instead of dividing the $38.5 million by 85,000 and getting something like $442.50, we divided the $38.5 million by 100,000 and the per pupil expenditure decreased to something like $385. I'm glad that we did this, however, because it really will emphasize to the legislature this year the seriousness of the legislation that they passed in the 87th General Assembly. Not many legislators really knew what they were doing when they passed this bill—a few did, of course. We're the only state in the Union that has moved in the direction of mandatory education for the handicapped without having a court order forcing us to do it. I think that is a credit to this state. The other possibility for stretching the funding this year, of course, is provided by the educational bill that has just been signed by the President. This could, depending on the amount of the appropriation, result in an additional $12 million which would be available to the state of Tennessee. With this $12 million on top of the $38 million, we would be getting pretty close to what we actually need for the implementation of this Act during this school year.

In addition to the services planned for local school systems, the development staff during the coming year will be engaged in several activities. (1) We expect to start the development of a comprehensive state plan for providing special education for corrective and supportive services to handicapped children by all state and local agencies. This is mandated in the Act. (2) We also must update the census report by requiring school systems again to look critically at the number of handicapped youngsters who reside in their school districts. (3) We must provide improved public information on the rights of handicapped pupils. We have started this by recently inserting an ad in every newspaper in the state informing parents of handicapped children of their rights. (4) We have to prepare an annual budget request based on the projected needs for the 1975-76 school year. Additional attention is being given to recommendations for change in certification standards which are appropriate for teachers of handicapped children. Attention is also being given to the due process provisions of the legislation and the notification of the public at large of the rights of handicapped children. The Governor, the Commissioner, the State Board of Education, and the Department of Education have recently been defendants in a civil suit which was filed by a group of parents here in Memphis on November 6, 1973. This suit alleged certain delays in implementation of the Mandatory Education legislation. A Consent Agreement was signed on July 19 of this year. The Consent Agreement settled all items in the original complaint which remained unsettled except for two pending issues. One complaint was that they wanted a division for the handicapped to be established within the State Department of Education and that this division be headed by an Assistant Commissioner. This has not been done because the department is now organized by functions to be performed rather than by segmented programs. If handicapped children are to be served in accordance with the legislation, the total organizational structure of the State Department of Education and the State Educational System must be respectively involved to that end. Significant progress has been made in establishing the framework for the Mandatory Education of Handicapped Children. The legislation which was enacted in 1972 is comprehensive and detailed. The General Assembly, our legislators, should be commended for enacting the legislation.

Let me stop here and review what is to be done in the future. This bill provides for a unitary educational system for all handicapped children in the state of Tennessee. At present time, we have the following state departments and the following people involved in the education of handicapped: Vocational Rehabilitation doing one thing for the handicapped and a Special Educational Component doing another thing. We have the State Department of Mental Health operating throughout the state several institutions that have an educational base. We have the State Department of Corrections operating educational institutions. We have private and public universities and colleges operating special education services. We have private organizations scattered throughout the state, most of which originated as a result of the interest of parents of handicapped children in coming together to form a school or a service for the handicapped. The big job that we have this next year is to pool all this together and come out with a sensible, coordinated plan for the education of handicapped children. The second big job that we have is selling educators on the idea that just because a child is handicapped doesn't mean that he's a second-class citizen. Now this is really hard to do. How do you convince school principals, school superintendents, and school board members that this child, this fifteen-year-old boy who is participating in your work study program, has the same basic rights as any other child within the school system? You say, "Oh, but goodness, we ought to already believe that," but we don't. I don't have to tell you people about this. You work with schools day in and day out, and you encounter ignorance as it relates to handicapped children.

Another aspect of the problem: this *least restricting alternative* must be observed in the placement of boys and girls in an educational program. We talk about mainstreaming, and people get frightened. "I don't want this mongoloid child in my regular first grade class." Everybody knows that mongoloid children shouldn't be in the first grade, and people become emotionally uptight, but we're talking about placing the child in a placement that is least restrictive *to him.*

This can be done. We have a system set up for the next school year whereby schools throughout the state will think in terms of four categories: A, B, C and D. Category A includes children, handicapped children, who are placed in regular classrooms and who need minimal assistance in order to achieve. This category might include children who need a special hearing aid. We would provide the hearing aids, then he would be placed appropriately, and that would perhaps be all that he would need. Category B would include the use of resource teachers. A child might spend a half day with a resource teacher and then be in the mainstream the other half, or three-fourths of the day with the resource teacher and the other quarter within the mainstream. Category C represents the conventional self-contained classroom. The plans that were submitted on July 1 from local school districts seem to indicate that most school systems throughout the state are complying with this concept of least restrictive alternative very seriously. Category D would include those children who need hospital and homebound instruction. During the year, every child in the state of Tennessee who is served in the program for handicapped children will be included in one of these categories.

We're trying to get away from labeling children with meaningless labels. With regard to identification and assessment of handicapped children, for years we have, in Tennessee and throughout the whole of the South and America, depended primarily on a psychological test. The psychological examination usually consisted of the administration of the Binet or the WISC and resulted in the magic score, the I.Q. We put that I.Q. number down and that became a label. If it happened to be less than fifty ,the child became known as a trainable mentally retarded child. From fifty to seventy-five, the child was labelled an educable mentally retarded child. And you know, it takes a good psychometrist just a matter of a couple of hours to determine what the label is going to be. In fact, we can completely label a child in a two-hour period of time, and then we spend the rest of his lifetime trying to remove that label. That's a strong adhesive that we use in putting the label on, isn't it? Somehow or other during this school year, we've got to make some progress in looking at the needs of children instead of trying to concentrate on labels that we've placed on children. I have a feeling that it would be possible to look at all children on the basis of their educational, social, health, and other needs instead of concentrating on a label that we've administered.

We have also anticipated some real problems related to serving severely handicapped children. We have set aside a sum of money within our allocation to provide what we call low incidence-high cost programs for children. We're talking about the deaf/blind child, the severely orthopedically handicapped child; maybe there are a half dozen or dozen different categories that we're talking about. Any school system has a right (not only a right but a mandate as a result of this legislation) to provide the service regardless of the cost. If we average out the $385 per child, we know that a number of the children who fall into Category A, or the mainstreaming category, won't require as much money as children in Category C, so the cost would average out. I signed a contract with a school system this week where next year the school system will spend $6,500 on the education of one child. It scared me because I know that we can expect the severely handicapped child to comprise as high as one-half of 1 per cent of the total school population. If the percentage is that high in the state of Tennessee and if we have to spend this amount of money on that number of youngsters, the cost will be exorbitant. But the legislation says that we must spend this money, so we've got a conflict. We've got the legislature passing an act that says you will do this, and the same legislature also has a responsibility for appropriating the money. So, in effect, how far we can go in the full implementation of this act depends on the amount of money we have available to implement. Not entirely, because I'm convinced that if we had $150 million right now we couldn't achieve the full implementation of this Act within the next five-year period.

Full implementation would depend on trained personnel—people who are really trained to implement this kind of program. The need is for teachers who have a broader outlook than those presently being prepared within our colleges and universities. We've got a lot of work to do there. We have a lot of work to do in reforming the attitudes of the educational professional within the state of Tennessee. We ought to be moving fast in this area. I guess we're still groping around. How do you really effect attitudinal changes? How do you get people who have said "deaf and dumb" all their lives to accept the fact that this is a misnomer? How do you really sell people on the rights of individuals, on basic human rights? Look at what has happened in the South since the Brown decision in 1954. We still have encrusted prejudices. They are eating away at us. And we have prejudices within the structure against handicapped children. So the job is a big one. The change won't happen overnight. But I think we can look at what has happened with a great deal of pride, recognize mistakes that we've made during the last year, and then look forward to the future of really implementing a program here in Tennessee that the whole nation can look at with a great deal of pride.

The $38.5 million that we have appropriated this year is not the whole story. This doesn't include the appropriation for the special schools like Tennessee School for the Blind and Tennessee School for the Deaf. It doesn't include monies that we're presently getting from the Federal Government under Title VI or Title II or money that we expect to get. I think that the state can be commended for the effort that has been made, but the job ahead is really staggering.

When the program that you represent was first initiated, I was in a pilot educational system in Chattanooga. The program was looked upon at that point as one answer among many alternatives in finding a way to help educate and place handicapped children in productive roles within our society; but it's not large enough. Now, the Mandatory Education Bill includes ages four through twenty-one. This range is going to give school systems a lot of concern. The bill still holds the school system responsible, even though a youngster has a diploma. Some people want to debate the issue, but the language is clear within the bill—age four through twenty-one. You know what that means. It means we're going to have to really do some planning for vocational placement of handicapped children, planning that we haven't done before. You can't wait until a boy or girl gets to be fifteen or sixteen to plan for vocational placement.

We've got a new term that is being bandied around in educational circles nationally, "career education." The term leaves me cold because I think we're talking about vocational education. I like to talk about vocational placement, and I like to see this process starting back at early identification and intervention with children. If we start at that point we can do intelligent planning. If we wait until this educable mentally retarded child gets into junior high school or high school, it's too late because attitudes are already formed. The youngsters lack skills, and then we start working our heads off trying to produce something that really can't be produced unless it is started much earlier. Let me stop here because I suspect that you might have some questions that you want to ask.

Question from the floor. I agree with the philosophy behind the bill that every student is entitled to education, but in thinking in terms of cost—right now the per pupil expenditure at the Tennessee School for the Deaf is $6000 per student; the breakdown on allocation is $385 per student—do you think we're ever going to have the funding to fully implement the bill, even if we had the personnel to do it? *Reply.* Yes, I think we're close to it right now, really, if you look at what is available. Remember, I am talking about state dollars only. In the education of children in Tennessee, we have more local dollars put into the educational budget than we have state dollars, so it might run as high as 60/40 or 65/35 of the local dollar. So you see, your big money is coming out of local dollars.

Question from the floor. In relation to special schools, such as the one I am associated with or facilities such as Green Valley Hospital and School, is this going to mean that those schools in the future might have to contract with local school districts for funds? *Reply.* This has not been resolved, but it is something we're working on right now. The concept of a local school district retaining responsibility for a child is a good concept, whether he's in the local schools within the district or whether he has to go outside of the district in order to get the services, because it holds one governmental body accountable for the child. I hope in the future that we can develop a system whereby the local school systems hold on to this responsibility and purchase services from institutions like Green Valley or Tennessee School for the Deaf, Tennessee School for the Blind, Clover Bottom, Arlington, or anywhere else. You know we have Tennessee Preparatory School operating in Nashville. Indigent, neglected children are committed by courts to TPS. Most of the communities that commit children to that institution have the attitude that it is no longer their problem, but this bill says it *is* their problem. I look forward to developing some kind of structure, some kind of system, that we can go through for the purchase of services with the funds we have available, and then supplement it with a state appropriation direct to the institution or to the appropriate department of government in order to do the job. I find that school systems are like people. If you put your money in the system, you're going to hold an interest. If you buy into it, you'll hold an interest, especially in children.

Question from the floor. The school you were speaking of in Nashville for indigent children: my experience has been that it's been for delinquent children. *Reply.* You're probably right, but the law says indigent and neglected children. It just happens that most of these indigent, neglected children really aren't adjudicated as delinquents. Delinquency is a legal term so they are not delinquents until they become adjudicated delinquents. The adjudication is on the basis of dependency and not delinquency.

Question from the floor. I just wanted to ask about the compulsory attendance law in relationship to this. Does this sort of supersede the compulsory attendance law and give the school authorities the legal responsibility until the individual is twenty-one so that the schools need to be doing something until then, or what? I know my question is not a very knowledgeable one. *Reply.* It's a very good question. In fact it's a question that we are wrestling with right now. The compulsory school attendance law was a law based on negative thinking. Probably the most cruel thing that the state lesislature has ever done is to require children to stay in school without adequate programs. We did this in Chattanooga. We went about beating bushes and bringing them in by the napes of the neck and placing them back in classrooms; and zip, out again. For eight years I operated a school for kids who were "kicked out" of regular junior high schools. We didn't have compulsory attendance at that school. We had programming for individual boys and girls, and, therefore, we didn't need compulsory attendance. I never did go out and beat bushes. This bill is saying you must provide a program, and the provision for due process says that if a parent isn't satisfied he can ask for a hearing and the hearing will determine whether the placement is satisfactory or not. This is good. All too long in education we've pretended we own the children. Kahlil Gibran, in his book, *The Prophet,* said, "These are not our children. They don't belong to us, they just pass through us." And I think that we're coming to the realization that we don't own these kids. Neither do the parents. They are children who have rights for appropriate placement.

Question from the floor. Now these hearings, in the case of parents' feeling that the child is not properly placed, the first echelon of hearing, I presume, would be with the local school authorities, school systems, and the last resort would be the lawsuit, I guess. *Reply.* The process works something like this. The parents of a child, who is in a school but not receiving the service that they feel he should receive, have the recourse to appeal to the principal of that school. If they don't receive satisfaction there, they appeal to the Board of Education. A hearing officer who is not a resident of the school district in which the case is located will be appointed. We have spelled out a set of criteria to be used in the selection of hearing officers. The hearing officer will go into the community and conduct a public hearing on this child—on the placement of one child. Fantastic, isn't it? You know, we're going to be inundated with appeals unless we start looking at what's happening to boys and girls, and I contend we should be.

Question from the floor. I have a comment. I anticipate one aspect of this bill that's really going to be good because the problem that we have with our city schools is that they have so many unqualified teachers, and these people are not certified in special education; we had five in one school this past year. They don't even know what to do if a child has a sort of seizure. Vocational rehabilitation is supposed to take care of a child in placement and all this, but they're finished with him, especially after they get in the twelfth grade; they're through with them. Some teachers take an interest and follow up, but the majority of them say, "Well, he's graduated now, I don't know if he's going to live or die." I think this bill is really good. It's going to make somebody get up or get out. They're going to do a good babysitting job. Let him sit down and learn to do something. *Reply.* I'm afraid you're right.

Question from the floor. Relating to what you were saying previously, I was thinking: are the school districts—you mentioned that several school districts were taking this least restrictive approach— do you think they are doing that because they feel they have a chance to implement that kind of program because of the costs as compared to Plan B or C or D that you were describing? *Reply.* In all fairness to school systems, I would have to take a very positive attitude toward them in regard to this and not try to determine what their motivation is, except to try to believe that they are doing it because they feel that this is the best way to serve kids. This system under which we are operating now makes it much more difficult to plan programs just to get money than did the old system. A lot of programs in the past were planned in order to increase the budget of the school district, and it worked that way. I see things differently now, but while I was in charge of this program in Chattanooga I was receiving reimbursement on one child from four different sources at one time. I was receiving four times what you'd normally receive because of loopholes in the rules and regulations in the law. I would hope that most school systems are doing it because they think this is the best placement for children.

Question from the floor. I'm really concerned because I think that in some cases the bill asumes that every classroom teacher has expertise in all the areas of special education categories, which isn't true at all. *Reply.* It also assumes that all classroom teachers are capable, qualified teachers, which isn't true at all.

Question from the floor. Earlier I noticed you mentioned that Vocational Education would provide services to all handicapped. We have an upper I.Q. cutoff score that we have to stay under. When the I.Q. falls below sixty, they're not eligible for vocational education. *Reply.* You see, this is part of the ambiguity under which we're operating. We have one group working to remove scores and labels. We have another group still putting them on. I was in Washington two weeks ago and I'm convinced that federal legislation is not going to stand in our way of removing labels. Now some little bureaucrats might, but the federal legislation is not going to.

Question from the floor. But students are still going to be grouped whether they are labeled or not. *Reply.* They are going to be grouped, but the important thing is why—to receive a specific service.

Question from the floor. Why has special education increased the pupil-teacher ratio from 1:15 to 1:25? *Reply.* This is a local thing, really. What they are doing is stretching dollars and watering programs. The truth of the matter is that we can't offer services of any higher quality to handicapped children than we are offering to normal children. In going from school system to school system throughout the state, there's a positive correlation between the type of program that is offered to the non-handicapped and the handicapped. If schools are doing jobs for non-handicapped children, they are doing good jobs for handicapped children, and the converse is certainly true. Dealing with youngsters is not an easy job, is it? It's hard. And I'm not naive enough to feel that the state legislature can mandate quality in education, but I wish they could. We wouldn't have some of these things happening. It is ridiculous to increase the per pupil ratio and at the same time expect program quality. Some teachers can serve fifty youngsters in some services. Some should be working with one child, you see. Any other questions?

Question from the floor. Why are they taking the vocational programs out of the schools? In Chattanooga they've taken all the shop and everything out. *Reply.* I happen to know about that situation. It's tied in with the court actions there of centralizing vocational work under one roof. I can remember when we were still training in Chattanooga in the vocational field, training boys and girls to do specific things that didn't even exist in job placement. We trained shoe repairmen down there, and the demand for shoe repairmen is very low, but we had twenty-five to thirty completing the program each year. We trained students to be tailors, a very popular offering because we happened to have two good teachers for these two courses, and a lot of kids took the courses. But we couldn't place them after they completed the program. By the way, one other thing I want to bring up and this has to do with records. This also relates to this bill. Parents have a right to see every record on their child. Parents have a *right* to see *every* record that is generated on their child; not just school records, but every record, including psychologicals. Attached to the educational act that has just been signed there's an amendment that spells this out even further, that a parent has a right to see any information that you have on a child.

Quesion from the floor. What does this amendment mean to us? *Reply.* You know what this is really going to do. It's going to make us act and behave in a professional manner. Instead of inserting unsupported opinions in records you must have something to back up what you say. If you use the word "'retarded" you've got to have some document in that record showing that an assessment, an evaluation of this child, indicates that he performs at a retarded level.

Question from the floor. What about talks we have with students where it has been agreed to keep it confidential between us? *Reply.* According to this, parents have a right to full knowledge of every record on their child. If you keep notes on your counselling sessions, then "yes."

Richard F. Bynum

The Need for Professional Education
in Disability Evaluation

The author is concerned with the improvement of the professional expertise of the disability examiner as well as his professional status. The basic concept behind professionalism is that of "public trust." This concept applies to the disability examiner in the same way it applies to the physician or lawyer even though licensing and legal responsibility are not required of the disability examiner.

Five characteristics which must be identifiable in order for a work group to attain professional status are listed with evidence that disability and evaluation meet these criteria. Emphasis is placed on reasons for the establishment and/or continuation and improvement of graduate programs in disability evaluation both for adequate training of new personnel and for upgrading skills of present examiners. Graduate education programs can make a significant contribution toward professional and personal growth.

I am very happy to have the opportunity to talk to such a distinguished group of disability examiners. You really are a special group of people because of the kind of work you are doing. Remember the first time you tried to tell someone what you did for a living? Not only is disability evaluation in and of itself a relatively new field of work, but also the fact that you are an employee of the state Department of Vocational Rehabilitation working under contract with the Social Security Administration is a concept that is difficult for most people to understand.

Your very notable efforts to assist quite a large number of Tennessee citizens who have filed disability claims during the past several months should be recognized. We have seen a phenomenal growth in the disability program nationally as well as here in Tennessee. With the steady increase in Title II disability claims and the initial number of Title XVI claims, the job of the disability examiner has not only become more complex, but also it has been subjected to the pressures of making decisions on this large number of claims within the shortest time possible. The records clearly show that the

Tennessee State Agency has done a remarkable job, and each and every one of you should be commended for his efforts. I know that the citizens of Tennessee greatly appreciate the extra effort and dedication to your work that you have so clearly demonstrated over the past several months.

In a recent issue of the *NADE Advocate* I was amused at one of the cartoons that depicted the disability examiner using a dart board as a decision aid. After seeing that joke, I could not help but wonder what kind of decision those of us would make who are not very proficient at throwing darts and who would perhaps miss the dart board altogether. Although it is fun to joke about the use of such a decision aid, I think all of us recognize that the decisions we render in the daily course of our work have a profound effect on the very lives of thousands of Tennessee citizens. The professional expertise of the disability examiner is the main issue to which I would like to address myself today.

During the past several years I have had the opportunity to talk with many examiners and supervisors from almost every state agency in our country. There exists a common concern for the improvement of the professional expertise as well as the professional status of the disability examiner. Universally, examiners, first-line supervisors, middle management, and agency directors have expressed a deep concern for upgrading all aspects of the disability examiner's professional life.

How can this be done? First of all, what are some characteristics of a profession? It has been suggested that five distinct criteria can be identified when a work group emerges into a profession: first, the establishment of a professional organization; second, the establishment of ethical practices and criteria for group membership third, the establishment of learning experiences and facilities directly or indirectly controlled by the group; fourth, legitimation of the group's monopoly over the services and activities performed; and fifth, development of an identity recognized and held by other professions, the public, and members of the group itself. On the basis of these five criteria it is apparent that disability evaluation is truly an emerging profession.

Before going on for a closer look at these five criteria and how they apply to disability evaluation, I would like to share some of my thoughts with you about the concept of professionalism and the notion of "public trust." Is the disability examiner really an advocate of the claimant? Congress legislated into existence a disability insurance benefit program of a compulsory nature. Citizens of this state and this country contribute to the Social Security fund involuntarily. As all of you are quite well aware the complexity of the program has grown tremendously since its inception in 1954, and average citizens do not have the knowledge, skill, or ability to process their own claims without some sort of assistance. Consequently, they are dependent upon the disability examiner to render, on their behalf, an equitable decision. In effect, they are trusting the disability examiner to properly adjudicate their claims and render the best possible decisions as quickly as possible. This involves the concept of "public trust."

This same advocacy position is relevant to a physician. Society has recognized that physicians have special knowledge and skill that the general public does not have. A sick person person seeks the advice and help of a physician because he possesses this specialized knowledge and skill. Society has established laws prohibiting individuals from practicing medicine unless they have proven themselves to possess this specialized knowledge and skill. In return, the physician has agreed to adhere to ethical practices, and all his activities are directed towards the patient's best interests. All of us then are in a position of trusting the physician when he gives us medicine, performs surgery, and renders other medical services, since we do not possess that specialized knowledge and skill to do it ourselves. This same concept holds true for a lawyer. He is the client's advocate in legal matters where the average citizen is unable to handle these matters for himself; hence, the notion of public trust.

Although the disability examiner does not undergo licensing procedures as do the physician and lawyer, the concept is nevertheless the same. The claimant is dependent upon the disability examiner to utilize the requisite specialized knowledge and skills in adjudication of disability claims. If the disability examiner is lacking in this specialized knowledge and skill and makes an erroneous decision either in the claims development process or in the final decision, this amounts to a breach of ethical practice. Although disability examiners may not be held legally responsible, as a physician in a malpractice suit might be, we are morally responsible to conduct ourselves in the most professional manner possible and render decisions on the basis of facts and evidence. In order to do this then the disability examiner must possess the basic knowledge and skills found within the field of disability evaluation and be constantly gaining new knowledge and developing new skills in order to keep pace with the ever increasing complexity of our program. The disability examiner has a moral and ethical responsibility to act as the claimant's advocate in adjudicating the liability claim.

Now that we have taken a look at the basic concept behind professionalism, let's take a closer look at the previously mentioned criteria or characteristics of an emerging profession. First of all, the disability examiners have a professional organization. Although not very old as organizations go, the National Association of Disability Examiners is growing both in number and in stature. As long as I can remember I have heard some disability examiners say, "What can NADE do for me? What do I get for my dues?" This perhaps would be an appropriate question if we were buying tickets to a play, or being forced into paying union dues, or being required to pay a vehicle inspection fee. I suspect that part of the reason this question comes up from time to time is that we are not exactly sure what purposes a professional organization serves. Each of us, I am sure, has his own views of organizations as such, but this is different from what a professional organization should be. Basically, it seems to me that a professional organization should be concerned with the professional activities of the members of that group and be concerned with improving these activities. Helping the disability examiner increase his or her expertise by improving adjudicative capability seems to me to be a fundamental reason for the existence of a professional organization. What you get for your dues is the opportunity to participate in activities directed towards improving your ability to do your job better. However, this requires the active participation of each and every member. It can not be achieved in a passive manner. I challenge each and every disability examiner to become active in his state and national organization, conduct research, write articles, and create forums and other meetings where important issues can be examined and discussed. Each member needs to take an active part in developing and improving the techniques of claims adjudication and in improving his own personal skills and knowledge. NADE provides a focal point, an organizational framework wherein these activities can take place. The very strength and benefits derived from an organization come from the members; it takes personal involvement on the individual's part to get his "money's worth."

In looking at the second criterion, it is evident that NADE has contributed to the establishment of ethical practices. This is outlined in our code of ethics. Also, group membership is further defined by the examiner certification procedures.

The third criterion is concerned with the development of specialized learning experiences and facilities. For years, this need has been met through inservice training programs held primarily in the state agencies. Many of these training programs have provided the examiner with valuable learning experiences. However, training is only one-half of the total process necessary for the development of the professional disability examiner. Simply stated, training is primarily concerned with "how to," and education is primarily concerned with "why." A graduate level educational program does not replace training but adds to the necessary growth and development of the individual examiner. It has been our sincere attempt to serve these educational needs these past few years at The University of Tennessee, Knoxville.

It might be of some interest to you that in June, 1974, we had our first four graduates receive their Master of Science degrees from our program. These graduates were Peggy Clements from Kentucky, Jim Smith from New York, Bill Flynn from Montana, and Ron Reed from Tennessee. We also expect to have quite a number of graduates receive their degrees during the coming school year.

I am sure that very few of you have ever had to go before a state personnel board or legislative subcommittee in an effort to upgrade the job requirements or obtain a pay increase for disability examiners within the state agency. Imagine with me for just a minute what this would be like. You have been asked to appear before a legislative subcommittee to present your arguments for upgrading the job requirements as well as for a pay increase for the disability examiners within your agency. You might first explain the monetary impact the disability examiner has on the state and national economy as well as the effect of his decisions on handicapped citizens. It has been estimated that each disability decision represents anywhere from $12,000 to $24,000 in possible benefits. Considering the average case load of each examiner, this would amount to the authorization of approximately $400,000 of Social Security trust funds per month, which is an awesome financial responsibility to undertake. Also, you might explain the impact the disability decision has on the lives of handicapped people and their dependents and that the average disability examiner makes hundreds of decisions each year.

Let us assume that you have presented one of the most convincing arguments that could possibly be made to support your request and that several of the committee members seem to be in favor of your proposal. At this point, it would not be unusual for one or two of these legislative committee members to express concern for the very responsible job that the disability examiner has and become curious about the educational requirements of those individuals who are currently engaged in this work. Questions are asked, such as "What are the educational requirements for hiring individuals as disability examiners?" "Since there are approximately 65 graduate education programs across the country for rehabilitation counselors, where are the graduate educational programs for the disability examiner?" These can be very embarrassing questions at this point, and I submit to you that the existence of graduate education programs for disability evaluation is absolutely imperative for the development of a recognized profession. They very lack of such graduate education programs would seem to support the contention that the disability examiner's job is really not at all that responsible and that your plea for upgrading the examiner's job and increasing his salary is just another bureaucratic maneuver.

The existence of graduate education supports the contention that we have a legitimate monopoly over the task of evaluating impairments and determining disability. This has always been an extremely difficult task and it is becoming increasingly more difficult as time goes on. The disability examiner must stay abreast of the changing medical, legal, and vocational factors inherent in disability evaluation. We have a legitimate monopoly on rendering these specialized services to handicapped citizens. This has been established through the Social Security Act, and there is no question but that the work requires a specialized body of knowledge and, most importantly, professional expertise.

If we are to expect the public and other professions to recognize and respect the profession of disability evaluation, the examiner must conduct his or her business in a competent and efficient manner.

Respect and professional integrity must be earned. Everett Hughes stated in *Men and Their Work* that "a profession is an occupation that has attained a special standing among occupations." Status, however, cannot be mandated or legislated; it must be earned.

The single most valuable resource to our national disability insurance program is the disability examiner. We must do everything in our power to nuture the development and growth of this most valuable resource. Ample opportunity for professional and personal growth must be provided if we are to foster the dedication and personal committment necessary to this complicated and responsible work. Graduate education in disability evaluation has been needed for many years, and, although we are just beginning to develop our program at The University of Tennessee at Knoxville, it is in the interests of all disability examiners, as well as all the citizens in this country, that we do everything in our power to ensure the continuation and improvement of graduate education for examiners everywhere.

Graduate programs in disability evaluation will encourage personal committment and dedication on the part of the examiner. As a practical result, turnover will be reduced and the quality of the ajudication process will be enhanced. The university campuses will provide a steady source of well-qualified examiners. It is true that many examiners working today got into this field because they happened to need a job, not because they felt that this was an important field of public service where personal and professional satisfaction could be achieved.

The existence of graduate education also helps in establishing the identity of the disability examiner and demonstrates to the public and other professionals that disability evaluation truly is a field that requires specialized knowledge and skills commensurate with a master's degree. Most importantly, the graduate education program will enhance the examiner's self-concept. Research in the behavioral science field has long since established the fact that one's self-concept—how we see ourselves in relation to others—determines to a great extent our performance. Robert Merton in *Social Theory and Social Structure* clearly indicates that the self-fulfilling prophecy concept can have a very profound influence on behavior. A survey recently conducted by the Bureau of Disability Insurance found that those students who attended the 10-week graduate course in disability evaluation at The University of Tennessee, Knoxville, had developed a better image of themselves and their self-concept was enhanced. This was also corroborated by the students' immediate supervisors in that it was observed that once back on the job these students approached the evaluation process with more confidence and more professional expertise than they did before attending the university. This is perhaps the best testimony one could have for graduate/professional education in disability evaluation.

Upon reviewing the five criteria that distinguish any work group as an emerging profession, it becomes very evident that the field of disability evaluation is rapidly moving in that direction. This presents a challenge to all of us who are concerned with rendering the best possible services to handicapped people. In fact, it is more than a challenge; it is really a mandate. Each and every one of us should begin to search for ways to increase his own professional expertise. No one else can do it for us; the responsibility is ours. Graduate education is an important part of this process. The continuation and improvement of formal education programs for the disability examiner will only materialize to the extent of your active interest and participation.

How important is your work to you and to the citizens of this country? How well prepared are you to serve as the claimant's advocate? These questions are basic to the professional growth of the disability examiner, and graduate educational programs can make a significant contribution toward this end.

Richard C. Chadwick

Disability Examiners

Cases involving denial of social security benefits because of disability may be appealed before the Administrative Law Judge of Hearings and Appeals. Approximately 45 per cent of these denials are upheld at this hearing level. Reasons for reversing denial decisions of disability examiners are explained. This explanation should be of special value to staff counselors with clients who are filing for benefits.

I am informed that you all are familiar with the Determination Process from the beginning of the application all the way through to the final decision of the secretary, so I'm not going into the technical phases or the procedural phases, only as they apply to this group and to me. On my recent tour of duty as acting member of the Appeals Council in the Bureau of Hearings and Appeals in Arlington, Virginia, I had the pleasure of attending the graduating class of a new group of special Administrative Law Judges who had just completed their training in the black lung program under the federal Coal Mine Health and Safety Act. Dale Cook, director of the Bureau of Hearings and Appeals, in his remarks to the graduates, stressed the ever increasing workload of those charged with the responsibility of making disability determination.

My purpose here today is not to remind you of the production pressures that you have had in the past and that administrative law judges have had, too, but to say that things will not get any better. We're all aware of and have often bemoaned the fact that in our work as government employees the primary emphasis has always been on the quantity of cases rather than on the hope or expectation of quality. In other words, they are always saying, "Get 'em out. Get 'em out." Whenever I hear someone say "There's one of those coffee-drinking newspaper-reading government employees," I always think how nice it would be to have the job that the guy thinks I have. So recognizing that you and I both realize that we have a tremendous job to do, I do not intend to bore you with a lot of statistics on past performance and projections for the future case load.

113

One statistic, I think, you *will* be interested in: that 45 per cent of your denials of benefits, nationwide, are allowed at the hearing level. I made a study of cases that I have decided, over 500 in my three and one-half years as Administrative Law Judge, and I find that I come to about the national average, give or take a few percentage points. Now, you may have thought that the Administrative Law Judge hearing a case obviously has some device by which he makes decisions, such as a lucky coin, or a dart board, and he has therefore substituted the fortuitous flip of the coin or a toss of the dart for your well reasoned good judgment, made following a thorough, microscopic search of the evidence before you, but this is not so. When we decide the case, we do have before us much more evidence than you had when you made your determination of the case. Let me give you an example. John Doe makes application for disability benefits under social security. On his application he states that he is no longer able to work because of back pain, and of course you've seen the application. This is the way they usually fill them out—just some little simple statement like that. The only evidence submitted in support of his claim is a short statement from a treating physician. I'm sure you've seen these, too, some of them on a prescription form. The statement reads: "To whom it may concern. I have been treating Mr. Doe for the past 18 months for low back pains. It is my opinion that he is unable to work." That's it. That's all you've got. But then to further develop the case you send a claimant out for a consultive orthopedic examination. Upon physical examination, the examiner finds that the patient can bend over and touch his toes, walk, walk on heels and toes without difficulty, and get on and off the examining table without difficulty; there are no muscle spasms or atrophy, no sensory, reflex, or circulatory deficits. X-rays of the spine show some mild degenerative changes, but the examining physician doesn't feel these to be significant. There is no evidence in the material before you that any other impairment exists. Sinec he has not alleged any other impairment—in other words, he hasn't said anything else about any other things that have bothered him in his application— the determination that you must make in the case is quite obvious. Mr. Moore did advise me that you all are familiar with the entire process, from the time of application up to the final determination; i.e., the decision of the secretary. Now, of course, in this process there is the initial determination made by you, the reconsideration, the hearing, the appeals council and then finally the appeals to the U.S. District court, if the claimant so desires.

During all of these processes, there is only one man in the process who ever actually sees the claimant, and that is the Administrative Law Judge at the hearing. The rest of the determinations are based merely on what we would call documentary evidence, or papers that you have in the files. You've never seen the claimant, and you know nothing about him other than what he says on his application. Now when he comes before the Administrative Law Judge for a hearing, he is questioned by the Administrative Law Judge. In addition to questions regarding his ability to stand and bend over and so forth, questions regarding his back pains, we also ask questions regarding other symptoms. In a great number of cases, this fellow may testify about his legs and back hurting, but he also says he has headaches, dizzy spells and shortness of breath, chest pains, and so forth. This then raises a question in the Administrative Law Judge's mind. Although there isn't any doubt about the fact that disability couldn't be granted based on an alleged orthopedic impairment, maybe there is something else that prevents this man from engaging in substantial gainful activity. So then we ask your agency to arrange a consultive internist examination. Now it may be discovered from that examination the guy has high blood pressure, cardio-vascular disease with enlarged heart, or some other serious condition. I think primarily this is the reason why your cases are reversed—because of the development that is brought out by questioning the claimant in the hearing. This also includes questioning of other witnesses; sometimes the claimant brings in his wife. Sometimes in the hearing you have a very inarticulate claimant who doesn't understand too much of what is going on, and you ask him whether there is anything else bothering him, either generally or specifically. You may ask specifically about headache and he will not give an answer that will give you any lead as to the possibility of other impairments. However, his wife says he complains about having headaches all of the time. So you can see that having the applicant before you does give you at least leads into further development that may be needed in the case, something that you, of course, in your process do not have the advantage of.

When we reverse cases, we don't only reverse you. We also sometimes reverse cases coming the other way. For instance, I had a recent case that went to the U.S. District Court in the western district of Tennessee, and the judge then remanded the case back to the secretary for further evidence, specifically as to whether or not the claimant's diabetes mellitus and high blood pressure could be controlled by medication. When I got the case I sent it out to an internist for an answer to those specific questions asked by the court. The internist in his report said that this fellow was very suggestible, that he answered, "Yes," to everything he was asked, and that he had a sort of a silly grin on his face all through the examination. All of this raised the question in my mind after the report came back as to whether or not there might be some mental impairment involved. So then I asked your agency to have a psychiatric evaluation made. The report came back that the fellow was operating at a very low level of intelligence, plus the usual thing that we'd need the listing, and we could allow a finding of disability based on a mental impairment. My recommended decision to the appeals council was therefore that the case be reversed. Incidentally, the internist found that the blood pressure was not elevated when he examined him and that the diabetes mellitus was controlled merely by diet without medication. You can see that, with answers only to the specific questions that the court had asked and had remanded the case for, there would have obviously been an answer in the negative. And it could have been that if we had confined ourselves only to that particular question without further development of the case, then, of course, the case would have been affirmed by the district court on going back to final decision; in other words, with only the new evidence then with the case that the court had required.

I think I mentioned that we are the first ones, the only ones, who see the claimant in the case. In his introduction, Mr. Moore alluded to the fact that I was an Assistant U.S. Attorney for twelve years. Now even at that level, the court level, although the claimant is the plaintiff in the case, the court does not take any new evidence; so, therefore, he doesn't appear. Cases before the U.S. District Court are handled on what we call the summary judgment basis; that is, the case goes up on the record that is made by the Administrative Law Judge, and the court decides then, based on that record, without taking any new evidence in the case, whether or not the decision was correct. So you see, the court—the U.S. District Judge—doesn't even get to see the claimant in the case. It has often been described that our job is one where we wear three hats; that is, we're a judge, we represent the claimant, and we represent the social security administration in the case. This is what makes our job difficult because I would say, although claimants on occasion do come in with attorneys, the attorneys usually are not all that familiar with the type of case that we are conducting, and they come in an adversary manner that they are going to have to fight somebody about getting the claimant's disability granted if he is so entitled. Of course, this is not the case.

Instead of following the usual procedure that a court would follow, that the plaintiff has the burden of proof so therefore he presents evidence first, I find that it is a lot more expeditious for me to ask questions of the claimant first and then let the attorney have him on "cross examination," This way I know what I want to develop in the case. I ask the questions that I think may bring out the points that I want to develop; whereas, if you ask an attorney or you let the attorney go first, he asks such questions such as, "Didn't you have an automobile wreck on such and such a date?" Of course I couldn't care less about how the disability came about. That's not an element in the case. All I am concerned with is whether or not the disability is there. It would make no difference to me whether the claimant had an automobile wreck or whether his wife hit him with a rolling pin. That doesn't enter into the case. So you find that a lot of time is wasted by attorneys trying to prove elements of a tort claims case rather than a disability case. In fact, I had one recently where the woman got a whiplash type injury in an automobile wreck and the attorney presented no less than ten different views of the automobile, which was totally wrecked. I admitted them into evidence and explained to the attorney that they had no probative value, but if he wanted to put them in the record, I'd be glad to put them there. And so I admitted them on that basis. That, of course, is one of the problems that we have in the hearings of these people.

Another problem we have is that the attorney may bring in twelve friends and neighbors to say that this claimant is disabled. Of course this testimony is really worthless. It has no probative value at all. It's merely an opinion of an unexpert witness. After about the third or fourth witness has testified, stating that he knows the claimant, has known him for ten years, knows that he's always been a good worker and knows that he's disabled, I always ask the attorney if the remaining witnesses will be just repeating what has already been testified to. If he so indicates, then I usually say, "I'm not trying to tell you how to run your case, and I'm not preventing you from putting anything in the record, but I think that there is really no point in cluttering up the record, making a long record with a lot of repetitive evidence that has no probative value." Usually they'll agree and won't put on any more of that type of evidence.

The other worthless type of evidence that you get from the so-called "character witness." That's the one who comes in and testifies that he knows the claimant, and he wouldn't tell a lie, and if he says his back hurts, it hurts. Of course you get maybe four or five people saying that type of thing, which again only clutters up your records. The integrity of the witness usually is not an issue in our case. If the man tells me he has a pain in his back, or if he tells the doctor he has a pain in his back, there's nobody who's going to make him say he doesn't have. What you do is try to find any medical evidence that will support his claim.

I've rambled on here for a few minutes now, and I hope that I have hit some highlights in what may be of interest to you, or what you may have wondered about as far as the Administrative Law Judge is concerned. I think, however, that perhaps I would be of better service to you if I allow you to ask questions now before we go one with any further statement of what administrative law judges do. With your permission, the floor is open to questions.

Question from the floor: When a claimant is being questioned during a hearing concerning possible medical problems, is there a doctor present? *Reply.* No. You just have to have a feeling about the thing. Sometimes you look at a guy and you know that he really has problems. You can tell by looking at him. Of course we can't decide the case based on what he looks like, but it does give us a lead, and of course we then would send out for a consultant examination.

Inaudible question. Reply: Most of the attorneys who represent these people at our hearing have represented them in a Workmen's Compensation case, and they feel like this is the same type of case, so an attorney comes in expecting an adversary type hearing. He gets the idea that I'm there to deny the case rather than to judge the case. Here's a good example, particularly these days when everybody is aware of individual rights. This case had the same element in it that this young lady over here asked about. The man's earning requirements expired in December, 1972, and he had a heart attack in

December, 1973, a year after. The only medical evidence in the file was that in August of 1973, before he had his heart attack, he had made application and they had sent out for a consultant's examination. He had two heart attacks, one on December 31, 1973, and one on January 1, 1974, and he kept insisting that he had a heart attack in 1973 and a heart attack in 1974, trying to indicate that it had been a continuing thing. Actually he was in the hospital at the time he had the second attack. At any event, he had a consultant examination in August of 1973. The attorney questioned the claimant extensively about when he had hired this particular attorney as his attorney and then in his legal argument he said that the claimant was sent out for a consultant examination when he didn't have an attorney, implying that somebody violated his rights, that he had a right to an attorney when they sent him out for an examination. The obvious question that I asked him was, "Well, do you think that would make any difference? Would it change the medical report in any way?" So I had to deny the case because I couldn't bridge the gap, couldn't get it back to December, 1972. Almost every day I have had a request to review his file, and when I do I'm sure there will be reference to the fact that the client didn't have an attorney when he was examined. What it has to do with the case, I don't know.

Inaudible question from the audience. Reply. No. You find them with all impairments; cardiovascular disease, all of them. If there is, I don't know about it. I have never actually sat down and made a study of it.

Inaudible question from the audience. Reply: There again I haven't checked any statistics, but I would say it would run about 70 per cent. We have a weekly report that shows the number of cases that are ready for decision and also shows the number for post-hearing developing. I would say that the figure runs about even; in other words, about the same ready for decision after hearing as there are; maybe about 50 per cent.

Inaudible question from the audience. Reply. I never request that the board certify specialists. Sometimes I request that a certain doctor not examine the claimant for various reasons. One, he may already have had a consulting examination by that particular physician, or the doctor may have at one time related to the client as his treating physician. Not using this doctor to examine him would eliminate any conflict of testimony. While we represent all parties, we feel like the doctor has to work with either one or the other. Now as far as the board certification is concerned, I think it is important if you have conflicting evidence where you have to give a greater weight to one medical report than to another, but we don't usually run into that particular situation. I don't think you would either, and, while in your cases you usually find differences of opinion, I don't think they are all that technical.

Question from the audience. Are you saying then that these requests usually are (inaudible)? *Reply.* Yes, there may be in the file conflicting testimony from two medical witnesses or medical documents that the judge can't resolve without a third, or another, examination. In that case he may want a more certified man so that he can say, "I have to select this man's opinion over that man's opinion because of his qualifications." But that's a rare case, I would say.

Inaudible question from the audience. Reply. Well, I wasn't aware of that. I don't know of any of the judges in our office who do. I just put a little note on the file, "Request internist consultive examination," and then it's usually sent to the state agency like that, unless there is some specific reason I don't want a particular doctor to examine the claimant. What the practices are in other offices in the state, I don't know.

Question from the audience: I'm aware that district courts are exceeding the authority that they have in reviewing cases. I can't be specific. I wonder if you would comment on the specific responsibilities or what the authority of the court is and how they may be giving the administration some problem in exceeding that. *Reply:* They are a reviewing court. They review the record and find whether or not the decision was based on substantial evidence in the record. I ran into this problem with a new judge when I was U.S. Attorney in Georgia. We had a new judge appointed to the bench. One of the first cases I had was a governor's motion for summary judgment in a social security case. It was a case where the claimant actually was not represented by council but had filed his own petition (which of course can be done in district court) and had come before the judge with motion for summary judgment. He had a hernia, and he told the judge that he had had a doctor tell him he had the biggest hole in his stomach that the doctor had ever seen. Well, I objected. I said, "Your Honor, there's nothing in the record that shows what he has testified to and the court is not permitted to take new evidence in the case. If the court desires new evidence, it can be remanded back to the secretary of HEW for new evidence, but the court cannot hear this evidence." I moved then to strike what the claimant had said. Being a new judge and being rather impressed with the guy trying to prosecute his own claim he said, "Well, I'll tell you what I'll do. Is the doctor who said that still practicing?" The fellow said, "Yeah." "Okay, I'll give you thirty days to get a statement from that doctor saying that you have the biggest hole in your stomach that he has ever seen." Thirty days went by and of course the guy couldn't come up with it.

This was a mistake that a lot of district courts make. While the evidence isn't really formally introduced, an attorney for a claimant may go before the judge and urge that the rejudgment not be granted based on the fact that there is new evidence to be had, resulting in the remand of the case. Once the district court was sitting in Jackson. Judge Welston was on the bench, and they were arguing some rejudgment in a social security case. Judge Welston turned to the Assistant U.S. Attorney and he said, "Has the earnings record expired in this case?" The U.S. Attorney said, "No, the claimant is still within eligibility." So then the judge turned to the attorney for the claimant and said, "Well, you know, she can file a new application," which impressed me very much because usually judges aren't all that sharp on this type of case. A lot of times somebody urges a procedure on them; for instance, in the case I referred to earlier in which the man was found to have a mental impairment, the judge remanded it for further evidence as to whether or not the diabetes and heart and blood pressure could be controlled. You look at the record in the case, and the questions are obviously answered. I think what the judge had in mind was probably urged upon him by the attorney for the claimant stating that his condition had worsened since the hearing. That was why, I think, the judge remanded the case. He would have been perfectly within the law to have affirmed the case rather than remanding it.

Inaudible question from the audience. Reply: We would like a large room, nice big bench, bailiff, a U.S. Marshal, and all the formality, but it's usually a very small conference room, particularly if we're out of our office area. The hearings are very informal, and probably rightly so, because if we did have the formality which is present in a regular courtroom, it might scare the plaintiff to death to come in there thinking that somebody is going to send him off for five years. In the informal setting, he doesn't feel so ill at ease. This is good because you have to drag everything out of many claimants anyway because they are very inarticulate. You have to use leading questions, and then what you have to do when you get your answer to the leading question is to determine whether he is saying "Yes" just to be agreeable or whether he is saying what is really bothering him.

Robert H. Couch

Vocational Evaluation of the Severely Disabled

Attention is presently being focused on services to the more severely disabled. Using the definition in the Rehabilitation Act as an aid in estimating the number eligible for such services, it is seen that present rehabilitation facilities can handle only a fraction of the possible cases. Other problems include the needs to educate the public as to available services and to change the current attitude of the counselor toward those clients with only marginal rehabilitation potential. Specific recommendations for improving services to this group are made, as well as predictions as to the changes that will come in evaluation tools, use of extended evaluation, job development, and job adaptation.

It is indeed a distinct pleasure to meet with you again in Tennessee. I congratulate you on the impressive and comprehensive conference program. I congratulate you also on the conference theme, Serving the Severely Disabled.

Some may say this new emphasis on the severely disabled is simply another in the long line of special disability groups upon which Washington has chosen to focus attention. Following this line of thinking, one might expect to wait until the emphasis shifts to another group. The demise of one disability group focus then would be quickly followed by another with little real change in client service programs. Some of you who work daily in rehabilitation facilities may well wonder who those clients you are working with now are if they are not severely disabled. Others are anticipating that clients in wheel chairs will begin rolling out of the wall in droves, thereby creating a new client population of middle-class intelligent, well-motivated individuals.

I suspect that none of these assumptions is entirely correct. The demand for services for the severely disabled will most likely endure; the severely disabled you serve now can and will be joined by those even more disabled; and you will find that many who happen to be confined to wheel chairs are also beset with problems of motivation, achievement, intellect, and social functioning.

As I have traveled throughout the region during the past few months, I have often asked counselors and facility personnel, "What are you actually doing with the severely disabled?" Unfortunately, the answer I hear most is, "Nothing much except emphasizing the severely disabled in meetings and talking a lot about it." In one state, a new counselor caseload was created especially for the disabled. Several experienced counselors were offered the new caseload, and all turned it down. These developments trouble me.

Thre are, however, a few promising signs. Tennessee's Smyrna project, Alabama's new Lakeshore Rehabilitation Facility, and the new V.R. involvement in Georgia's Warm Springs Foundation offer better services for the severely disabled. Previous performance in serving the severely disabled was a criterion for promotion for counselors in at least one Tennessee area. No doubt there are other movements of which I am unaware, and we can expect many new innovations with the severely disabled in years to come.

But just who are the severely disabled? How many are there and where might they be found? The Rehabilitation Act has defined these, and they inevitably include the blind, the deaf, the spinal cord injured, the retarded, the mentally ill, stroke victims, the alcoholic and drug addict and the epileptic. Most certainly there are others because the severity of a disability is relative.

In Tennessee's ninety-five counties, stretching for several hundred miles from the banks of the Mississippi River to the Great Smoky Mountains, there are almost four million people. Taking some of the standard estimates of incidence of disability, we might get a rough idea about the magnitude of this special severely handicapped population in Tennessee. We may find some 6,000 non-institutionalized adults confined to wheel chairs and another 34,000 severely physically handicapped individuals. If the 3 per cent estimate of retardation is accepted, we might expect up to 60,000 mentally retarded adults in Tennessee. No less than 100,000 adults would be found with emotional problems needing attention. Two thousand deaf individuals would be expected, and another 10,000 adults would exhibit hearing problems. Twenty thousand adults would exhibit total or partial blindness, and almost 100,000 would exhibit problems with alcohol. All together, upwards of 300,000 individuals might be found in Tennessee who have severe physical or mental problems. There are 300,000 severely disabled Tennesseans, and we boast of our record of rehabilitating just over 300,000 individuals in the whole country last year.

Suppose we attempted to serve just one half of the severely disabled in Tennessee. Could your Rehabilitation Facility handle its 4,000 clients? How would you handle your proportional share? If we only served one fourth of the severely disabled in our facilities, could you handle 2,000 severely disabled clients? Only serving a meager 10 per cent would mean at least 100 clients per facility; and few, if any, of Tennessee's facilities handle that many clients today.

So, realistically, what can we do to prepare to serve the severely disabled in facilities? First, we must locate these individuals and let them and the public know what rehabilitation is all about. People are, for the most part, ignorant of the fact that rehabilitation programs even exist. If you don't believe this, walk down the street of any city in Tennessee and pick out, at random, ten people. Ask them what vocational rehabilitation is and what services it provides. Unfortunately, I suspect not more than two in ten are even aware of rehabilitation. You and I know that rehabilitation facilities provide services for the severely disabled. I believe that vocational rehabilitation must advertise heavily to educate both the public and the handicapped citizen. If our services and our product do not merit public awareness as much as some of the heavily advertised deodorants and soap powders that are household words, we may as well give up.

Second, we must help break the response set of V.R. counselors who, because of heavy work loads, tons of paperwork, inadequate funding, and demand for "twenty-six closures," fail to pay adequate attention to those who need their help the most. Counselors train themselves to turn down or ease out the severely disabled and learn to do this with a clear conscience. Current procedures, demands, resources, and methods of measuring counselor merit have forced the rehabilitation counselor to adopt his current *modus operandi* so that he can actually sleep well at night after have turned down an individual who, admittedly, offered only marginal rehabilitation potential.

Now this is no "ivory tower" college professor conjecture. One state in this region studied referrals made to Vocational Rehabilitation and found that fully 52 per cent of those individuals referred did not make it into a rehabilitation category. Something is wrong, and I wonder what that rate is in Tennessee.

When beginning as a rehabilitation counselor, I was taught, unofficially of course, how clients could be eased out. These techniques and measures were resorted to by many counselors, not because they were lazy or non-caring but simply as a means of surviving. Racing to meet closure quotas, answering thirty calls daily, interviewing nearly forty people daily and attempting to prepare the required five pounds of paper documentation weekly precluded any real concentration on innovative and time consuming aid to the severely disabled.

This subsequent learned "response set" to the severely disabled must be broken if successful work with the severely disabled is to become a reality. Our own V.R. family attitudes and practices must be overhauled, and those of us in the facility movement can work for these necessary corrections. You can seek new and innovative services that can facilitate the work of the counselor, seek recognition for those counselors who do serve severely handicapped individuals, and advocate better ways of keeping score than the current "twenty-six closure" system. Congress has been clear in that they want us to change our ways!

Third, you must learn about the severely disabled, their special needs, precautions, and functional limitations. Take courses at your local universities that can enhance your competencies. You can attend training programs such as this one and others that no doubt will become available. Read first-person accounts written by individuals with severe disabilities to gain insight into their problems and perceptions. The professional literature abounds with articles relating to disability, and we must inform ourselves.

You must also get your own house in order. A highly trained evaluator and counselor in each facility is mandatory. Most Tennessee facilities are grossly lacking in this highly important area. How are the transportation facilities to and from your facility? Is your facility truly accessible to the handicapped? If you do not now have a medical consultant you should secure one skilled in handling severe physical problems. Many Tennessee facilities are not accessible due to architectural barriers within the facility itself. How can we hope to serve the disabled when they can't get into our facilities and use them? Has your facility legally complied with OSHA standards which ensure that your clients are safe within your building? Concrete steps to overcome many deficits noted in Tennessee facilities must be taken if you are serious about working with the severely disabled.

The vocational evaluation process is essentially the same for all individuals regardless of ability or disability, and few special evaluation techniques have been developed exclusively for the severely disabled as a group. Adaptations in testing the blind and deaf are well known, but those too coincide with the evaluation process.

A highly skilled evaluator is a prerequisite for evaluating any disabled person. Vocational Exploration for those forced to change careers will likely be a more popular and relevant evaluation tool. Utilization of physical and occupational therapy consultants may be commonplace, and full utilization of the currently available extended-evaluation will become standard practice in our work with the severely disabled. Job development and job adaptation will become a bigger area as ergonomics and other industrial engineering practices will be needed to make jobs accessible to the severely physically handicapped.

As we explore and experience work with this special group, new methods will evolve. I welcome this new emphasis and trust that together we can do whatever is necessary to ensure that the severely disabled have every access to the resources of our society.

Robert H. Couch

The Vocational Evaluation and Work Adjustment Association

The history of this association is given beginning with its origin in Georgia in 1965. VEWAA is described as an action-oriented, "do-something" organization formed for professional stimulation. Its general purpose is stated to be promotion of high ethical practices in vocational evaluation and work adjustment training of the handicapped. Encouraging the development of professional training opportunities and promoting research in the field are other purposes. "Mini-grants" are available for research projects.

I want to congratulate you on the formation of the Tennessee Vocational Evaluation and Work Adjustment Association. With the awarding of your charter, Region IV becomes the first region in the nation to have a state VEWAA unit in every state.

I want to talk to you briefly about your association, its origin and history, and your role in your professional organization. Consider these questions: What can VEWAA do for me, and what do I get for my money? What do I have to offer, and what does VEWAA offer me? What is VEWAA? What does it mean to me in my own professional work?

Back in the late sixties, a group of evaluators in Georgia often experienced times in which they stayed home and worked as they watched counselors, supervisors, and others go off to conferences. When their colleagues returned, they heard stories of the good times and the professional stimulation. They were somewhat jealous. They felt isolated. They felt left out. They worked daily in their evaluation units and oftentimes wondered, "Am I doing this right? What is it I'm supposed to do?" In their isolation they perceived themselves in a cocoon. So these people in Georgia back in the sixties felt this way. They asked, "Why can't we have an organization like the counselors and some of the other groups do? Why can't we get together? Why can't we fight this isolation and this stagnation and share our knowledge and concern for our profession and for handicapped people in

129

facilities?" I think this would probably sum up the way I perceive that they felt. So evaluators like Bill Baker, Frank Kern, Horace Dennis, Bodie Brown, Henry Mitzner, Bill Rabucca, Jim Perry, and others complained, they worked, and then offered an alternative.

Through the efforts of these individuals in Georgia, the American Association of Work Evaluators was organized in 1965. They met a couple of times just with Georgia evaluators. All of a sudden people from other states wanted to belong. Others had felt this isolation and they joined. While it was not a very large organization, they got inquiries from California, Iowa, and Wisconsin, and the interest stemmed from this need for professional stimulation. At one of the first annual meetings, I still recall reading that the late Gordon Haygood, who was a great influence and had a great impact on facilities of this region, when he spoke to this first organized group of the vocational evaluators in Georgia, said, "I have a feeling that this is the beginning of something great." We have lived to see something great come out of this. As a result of these efforts, the National Rehabilitation Association in 1966 organized an ad hoc committee to study the feasibility of a professional division within NRA. Dr. Paul Hoffman was selected as the ad hoc committee chairman. Through the efforts of Hoffman and others a monumental effort began to get the organization off the group. In 1967, I believe it was, the division was given professional status by NRA, and in 1968 full ranking national status as a professional division within NRA was achieved.

Few professional divisions began with such enthusiasm as was evidenced by VEWAA members. Everywhere, VEWAA members were excited about their profession. They were excited about their organization. In Alabama today, VEWAA is the largest professional division in the state. A year or so ago an NRA official said of VEWAA, "Your enthusiasm and your movement and your professional interest have created such a big stir that we're losing lots of our other divisions' members to VEWAA. It's such an action-oriented, 'do-something' organization." It's embarrassing now to think about how few resources we had. But we borrowed from any and every source we could find. We hitched rides, and we went to meetings, and we got organized, and we got some things going.

But what do you get from VEWAA? From a tangible type of basis—not really a whole heck of a lot. You will get a membership card and a certificate, and if the NRA computers don't mess up, you will get the *Journal of Rehabilitation* and the *VEWAA Bulletin*. But when you think about being a pioneer in a new field, it's very exciting. I'd rather pioneer in a new profession than associate myself with a very established professional group in which I have little impact or input. You too have this opportunity. As a VEWAA member you get on mailing lists, and in turn new doors open for you to get information from the outside on what's going on in the field.

I'd like to look for a moment at some of the purposes of VEWAA. When we first considered organizing an Alabama unit someone got up at our ad hoc meeting and said, "Look, if we're going to have an organization, that's all right, but I am not going to join another 'do nothing' organization." So we made a commitment at that time to be involved and to do something and have a "do something" organization rather than just one of these once-a-year get-togethers where we only sit down in a meeting and then go back and forget about it for a year. We planned to do something. So our group sat down and said, "Let's look at the purposes of VEWAA. From this, let's see what we can do ourselves to fulfill these purposes." We found that if you get something from VEWAA it's going to cost you more than $5. It's going to cost you your time, your commitment, and your interest. If you are willing to pay this price, then you're going to get a heck of a lot from your membership in your organization.

Our general purpose is promoting the highest ethical practices in vocational evaluation and work adjustment training of the handicapped. In the last few years, we've had a national VEWAA project which concides with this purpose. In this project local VEWAA forums were organized across the nation to ask some of the basic questions about our standards and practices. This input came from the field rather than from the top because you are the ones who are there and know what's going on. I attended one of the conferences synthesizing the input from sixty of these forums held in the country. VEWAA brought a group of professionals together down in Atlanta for this task, and I tell you I have never worked so hard in my life. We put in twelve to fifteen hours a day and had people going all night long at the typewriters. But it was one of the most exhilarating professional experiences I have ever had. Here, people were speaking to us from the field: "This is what we believe, this is what we think, and we want you to listen to us." This is what VEWAA really is. We also have in our association a code of ethics. You can be guided by these ethical principles in your work with other people because we're charged with guiding life directions for other humans, and that is no light matter.

Promoting and encouraging the developing of professional training opportunities for persons engaged in vocational evaluation and work adjustment training for the handicapped is another VEWAA purpose. This has been one of the most exciting aspects. The program that I am with in Auburn and the development of the program at Stout State, although they had other origins, came partially from VEWAA members. What may be even more exciting in staff development and training is this idea of the VEWAA Forums which people have developed in several of the states. Through these local forums, people who are working get together and train themselves, saying, "Look what I did last week; look what I found that works."

Encouraging and promoting research in the field is another purpose. Now, to begin achieving this purpose another one of those brassy VEWAA ideas was necessary. You know it is somewhat presumptuous to award research grants when you have 2,000 members and only $5,000 in the treasury, but VEWAA decided to start a research program. So we started the VEWAA mini-grant program. If you want to do a little something in the area of research, norm a work-sample, research the literature maybe, or need to do a master's or doctoral thesis, VEWAA might be able to help out a little financially. This is something you as an individual, you as a facility staff, or you as a state unit can do in the area of research.

So what can you get from VEWAA? Anything you want. But it's going to cost more than the $5 you put into it. You can sit back and do absolutely nothing, come to a meeting once a year, or you can get out and create and innovate and do anything you want. If you have a problem, a professional problem, that needs to be worked on to enable you to serve better handicapped people your organization can and should do something. It is not going to do it for the $5 you spend, but if you are willing to spend much more than the $5 in your own time and commitment, there is absolutely nothing that you can't accomplish through your professional organization. I want to keep an eye on the Tennessee VEWAA. I want to see it grow and prosper professionally.

The Vocational Evaluation and Work Adjustment Association, Present and Future

As his term as president of VEWAA nears an end, Mr. Gaines reviews improvements made in the structure of administrative practices in the organization and in the communication mechanism. He emphasizes the need for awareness on the part of the elected officers and the executive council of their responsibility and accountability to the members of VEWAA.

VEWAA has the important role to play of advocate on behalf of evaluation and adjustment practitioners in areas of reclassification, upgrading, and comparative salary schedules. Other matters of concern to VEWAA include the placement of more emphasis in the area of work adjustment and the advocating of more inservice training programs and training opportunities for practitioners.

Thank you for your very kind introduction. I'm not going to read all of this material I've brought to the podium with me, but l will refer to some of it during the course of my remarks.

I don't relish following Bob on the agenda because of the very fine job he did. His was an excellent account of the progress VEWAA has made during the few years of its existence. I particularly appreciate his remarks about what VEWAA offers its members and its basic purposes. This moring I wish to offer you some insight into VEWAA as it is now and what the future might hold for the organization.

This year, during my term as President and during this current Executive Council's tenure, we have dedicated ourselves to providing more definitive structure to VEWAA's administration, primarily in the officer ranks and in the setting of objectives for work to be performed in the association. More importantly, we have addressed ourselves to those ways we might become more responsive and realize in a more vital manner our accountability to you, the membership of VEWAA. As elected officers of the association, we've spent a substantial amount of time and effort in attempting to structure ourselves in order that we know precisely what we are to the association and, in essence, what we should be doing.

We've set into motion this year an objective setting planning process which will allow VEWAA officers henceforth to set objectives and develop an annual work plan at the beginning of the membership year. If you've read the last two issues of the *VEWAA Newsletter*, you will recall that the Executive Council has reported in that publication those goals it has set for this year and ways in which it will follow through. Publicizing this particular information is a measure we feel is important to the membership. As Bob pointed out during his presentation, people have often asked, "What's going on in VEWAA?" People have complained about not knowing what's going on and have wondered what the national officers were doing. The Executive Council felt that reporting its goals, activities, and plans via the *Newsletter* would be the best method to keep the membership apprised of what has been done, what's going on, and what has been planned.

In attempting to structure the administration of VEWAA, because, again, we do want to be more responsive to our membership and demonstrate our awareness of the need for responsiveness and accountability, we've tried to use a basic model of Management by Objectives (MBO) in establishing an annual work plan for the association.

The Executive Council met in Washington, D.C. last February and, so far as we know, it was the first meeting the Executive Council of VEWAA has been able to conduct in a face-to-face situation other than at the annual National NRA Conference. Theretofore, communication pertaining to plans, projects, or whatever had been conducted by correspondence, but in Washington we had the opportunity to convene and plan more effectively. We reviewed and discussed several tasks recommended by both members at large and members of the Executive Council. We tried to assess the association's state of the art and what was needed. Through that brainstorming session, we established several goals for this year and, thus, our work plan.

Another significant effort this year has been our attempt to gain more voice and become more active in the activities of the National Rehabilitation Association. I'd like to talk about this a little more later on in this presentation.

In setting our work plan into motion, we have appointed chairmen to various committees, and we have done so with some basic expectations. For example, each committee will be chaired by a person selected by the President; each committee will be comprised of a specific number of people selected from the membership at large by the President and/or a particular committee's chairman; each project to which a committee is assigned will have a completion date set; each chairman will be responsible for preparing a narrative report to the President at the conclusion of his or her committee's efforts. That project report is to describe the efforts that led to the project's completion and the project's outcomes. This is felt to be a beneficial measure to keep people on their toes, and it does make clear the accountability I mentioned previously. Through this approach, we can report to the membership in a more definitive manner.

Now, back to our effort in the area of NRA activities. As Bob pointed out, VEWAA is small in numbers, but loud in voice. Actually, I believe we are now the second largest division in the National Rehabilitation Association. Too, I believe that because of our overt attempts to maximize efficiency in the running of this association's business, we have made some favorable impacts in the NRA. I feel that the leadership in VEWAA has indirectly lent itself to some very positive improvements in the National Rehabilitation Association during recent years. However, at this point in time, we have failed, through direct dialogue, in getting the NRA to straighten out its membership program problems. For example, let me ask the question, "How many of you have failed to receive your VEWAA publications and how many of you have not been credited with having paid your 1974 membership dues?" Let me go on record as having stated that this is not VEWAA's fault! NRA, as you may or may not know, has its own in-house computer system now and has had this system for about nine or ten months. We have been told repeatedly that the membership reporting and mailing problems would soon be history. But alas! the problems persist, and we persist in keeping NRA aware of the persistence. So, again, please understand that, although we are not immune from making mistakes, the mail and membership problem does not originate in VEWAA. When you fail to receive a publication or you are not credited with having paid your dues, don't hesitate to let us know. We'll make every effort to straighten the problem out with NRA and see that it doesn't happen again. We all look forward to the momentous occasion when these problems do, in fact, become history.

Bob talked a bit about the states of Arizona and Georgia and about the advocate's role national VEWAA took in behalf of evaluation and adjustment practitioners in those states as well as in other states. Let me briefly mention something that happened in my own state, North Carolina. During my term as President-Elect, the State Personnel Department in North Carolina acted in behalf of our requests that the Vocational Evaluator positions be studied so that, hopefully, reclassification and upgrading would result. What we were really in hope of was that the Evaluator position would be classified at least commensurately with the Rehabilitation Counselor position. At that time, the Evaluator was at a salary grade four levels below the Counselor. For emphasis' sake, we verbalized that the Evaluator should probably be one step above the Counselor level. Anyway, as this study was beginning, I wrote a letter to Chuck Smolkin, who was President of VEWAA at the time. I informed him of the study and I requested that he write a letter to the Director of our State Personnel Department similar in content to the letters Bob described as having been sent the governors of Arizona and Georgia.

I asked Chuck to include in his letter some information about comparative salary schedules in other states with respect to Evaluators and Counselors, and I asked that he cite the need for the equalization of pay as based upon academic expectations, experience, and role responsibilities. Chuck wrote the letter and the Director of State Personnel had it three days after Chuck had received my request. I received a copy of Chuck's letter so that I would be in a position to discuss it if called upon by staff in the personnel department. The letter was very forthright and, in essence, appealed to the State Personnel Department's sense of fairness. To make a long story short, I received a telephone call from the State Personnel Director's office, and the caller wanted to know, "Who in the hell is Chuck Smolkin?" and, "Where does he get off writing such a letter?" I explained that he had been requested by me to write the letter because of our national concern about the inequitability in the salary schedules for Evaluators and also became I didn't think a letter from another North Carolina state employee would have the impact that Chuck's letter would. I got the distinct impression from the caller that Chuck's letter didn't carry too much weight, and I got the further impression that it would probably take something akin to an act of Congress to have any impact with that caller. The study was conducted and completed and the result was somewhat "middle of the roadish." Evaluators in North Carolina were reclassified to a salary grade one step below counselors, but a new position was established. We now have a Chief Evaluator, a position classified at one step above the Counselor level. The problem with this position is that there have to be at least three evaluators under the supervision of an evaluator before he or she can receive the "Chief" classification. We just don't have an abundance of facilities or programs wherein we have that many evaluators.

I've talked about the North Carolina situation with you to emphasize the point that national VEWAA can play an important advocacy role for its practitioners. Although we weren't as successful in North Carolina as we wished, we have been in instances such as the efforts described in Georgia and Arizona. I believe this kind of role should expand in the ensuing years in VEWWA, and for it to do so members are going to have to call on the national office, the Executive Council.

Another matter to which we have dedicated ourselves as officers this year is proper placement of more emphasis in the area of Work Adjustment. It has become obvious in recent years that we have devoted most of our attention to Vocational Evaluation and have, in so doing, given only lip service to Work Adjustment. At the very least, we are going to work toward an equalization of emphasis in Vocational Evaluation and Work Adjustment.

Just to give you an indication of our efforts of emphasis in Work Adjustment, let me mention a project we have in the mill. As you recall, Bob mentioned a bit about our current Evaluation Project, and he mentioned the Atlanta workshop. I just happen to have with me this morning a report dealing with the outcomes of that meeting. If nothing else, we're going to benefit the International Paper Company tremendously, considering just how much of their product we have used and will be using through the completion of the Evaluation Project. To back up what I'm saying about increased emphasis in Work Adjustment, we have established a committee to be chaired by Tom Gannaway which will have as its task the drafting of a grant proposal for funding of a Work Adjustment project similar in design to our current Evaluation Project. The proposal will be submitted to the Rehabilitation Services Administration via application for funding. This committee is to complete its final draft and submit it to the Executive Council for review and subsequent action at the annual NRA Conference in Las Vegas in October.

Our Pacific Coast Regional Representative, Dr. Fred McFarlane of San Diego State University, has written a project proposal for a short-term training program in Work Adjustment Services. The proposal and its grant application have already been submitted to the Rehabilitation Services Administration, and we expect word any day now regarding a decision. We are very optimistic about its possible approval. What we would like to use this project for is to "springboard" ourselves into the long-term project that Tom Gannaway's committee is working on. We would use the short-term project to establish an outline of work, the pattern in which we would conduct a three-year Work Adjustment study, and then begin the project as soon as the Evaluation Project expires. So we are getting more involved in the area of Work Adjustment and it's certainly high time that we did.

Another thing VEWAA should do, and will begin doing from the national level, is advocating more inservice training programs and opportunities for practitioners. North Carolina's VEWAA Chapter cited the need time and time again to the Vocational Rehabilitation agency for inservice training for evaluators and adjustment practitioners and, in a measure, it's paid off. Up until this past year, training for evaluators and adjustment practioners was almost nonexistent. We have the Regional program at Auburn for Evaluators, but that's it. Vocational Rehabilitation in North Carolina structured a forty-four week curriculum in evaluation and adjustment for practitioners in that state, primarily as a result of the VEWAA chapter's constant input. The results of that curriculum cannot be measured yet because the first cycle is not yet completed. But, here's an example of what VEWAA can be instrumental in doing. Left alone, North Carolina Vocational Rehabilitation would probably have eventually developed something for evaluators and adjusters, but credit is due the VEWAA Chapter for perhaps expediting the action. You can do it too! We should all be concerned with the lack of relevant training opportunities, and we shouldn't be hesitant to be heard. Brash? Bob used the word earlier. Damn right we should be brash if that's what it takes. People generally don't listen if not spoken to and oftentimes not even then. Sometimes it takes a brash approach, but that's all right. Issues have to be raised, and often repetitively, until resolution is achieved. We need more training programs and we are not, obviously, going to get them unless we cry out.

The Executive Council wants to hear from you. We have invited you to communicate with us, and we have publicized that invitation in every publication the association has. If you've got a problem, a gripe, a concern; if you want to praise somebody; if you've got a recommendation, suggestions, let us know. We don't discard input from our members; we use it. In a major sense, our work plan this year was developed from membership recommendations.

As I said earlier, the primary purpose for including work plan related information in our *Newsletter* is to keep the membership apprised of activities in the association. What we are really doing through that medium is saying, "Here's what we are doing now. What else should we be doing?" It's your obligation to respond to that invitation when you want to be heard. Too, it's not nearly so valid now for members to complain that they don't know what's going on and that they don't have a voice. We are going to keep you informed, and we ask you to consider how you can help us to continue to foster growth and meaning in our association. Without any reservation, I will state that this association offers its members a mighty fine dividend for an annual $5 investment. Ours is a strong organization principally because of the strong dedication and interest of its members.

Let me talk for a few minutes about the Rehabilitation Act of 1973 and its implications with respect to rehabilitation facilities and, ultimately, to VEWAA. The role of rehabilitation facilities, from the smallest to the largest, most sophisticated, is going to have to become more diverse and proficient. The emphasis proclaimed in the new legislation, services to the more severely disabled, will have its ultimate impact in the rehabilitation facility. The role, those services offered in the facility, is going to be magnified as never before, and the role of the evaluator and the adjustment practitioner will be in the limelight that much more. These practitioners are going to be relied upon more and more as the federal regulations resulting from the new legislation are implemented and the accompanying expansion of services to the severely disabled is realized. VEWAA is going to have to address itself even more constantly to the need for ever improving services in evaluation and adjustment, and it's going to have to gear itself to do a more intensive job of advocating and enhancing the growth, professionally and financially, of the practitioner's role. What I'm saying is that we have an opportunity not only to enrich the lives of severely disabled people, but we also have an opportunity on the horizon, I believe, to enhance and enrich the lot of our practitioners through the increased expectations of and services delivered by evaluators and adjusters.

It is my personal hope that this association will assert itself in behalf of its members as we progress into the new era opened by the Rehabilitation Act of 1973. In Tennessee, one person might not be able to accomplish much in the advocacy role, but as a common cause chapter you might. I encourage you to call on me or any of your other officers in this association if and when you believe we can assist you in your goals in this state.

In conclusion, let me briefly summarize the important issues I have touched on this morning. We have tried to streamline the administration of this association this year and included in that streamlining is a better communication mechanism. We believe we now have a structure which will better accomodate future growth in the association and which will allow for maximal membership involvement. We seek your input, we'll use your input, and we know we'll be a stronger organization because of it. Sooner or later, and sooner we believe, we'll see NRA get its membership mess straightened out and we'll all be happier as a result.

My term of office expires in October. I wish to thank you sincerely for electing me to this office and for giving me the opportunity to serve and increase my knowledge of evaluation and adjustment services. You have an excellent chapter here in Tennessee, and you are to be commended for your interest and your activities. It's because of you and people like you that we have a good organization. As long as our membership maintains interest, involvement, and dedication such as yours, VEWAA will continue to grow and be a dynamic and meaningful unit. Even with all of the NRA computer problems we've had in the membership program this year, we have grown by at least 15 per cent. It's a job well done, and it speaks well for all of you. Thank you for inviting me here, and I have enjoyed this conference very much.

Arnold B. Sax

Adjustment Services for the Severely Disabled

The goal of the adjustment program is to identify and modify problems which hinder the severely disabled in becoming contributing members of society. Such problems are not unique to any one group. Dr. Sax suggests that the interests of everyone would be better served with a program that would seek to identify needs common to all handicapped persons, and that would include provisions for special delivery systems to meet individual needs. Goals would be the development of pragmatic, functionally operative programs and the training of persons in the proper use of those programs.

Important concerns in working with the severely disabled are those of attitudes and expectations of the staff working with the client and the need to develop the client's independence, motivation, and realistic expectations. Materials are currently available for use in the development of adjustment programs.

The topic I have been given to discuss this morning is Personal Adjustment for the Severely Disabled. With your indulgence, I wish to broaden this topic and also include social and work adjustment for the severely disabled.

Our goal in rehabilitation is assisting the individual to become a contributing member of society. We need to identify the individual's problems that hinder his being able to become a contributing member of society. Our goal in the adjustment program then is to modify, change, or train the individual in such a way as to lessen these problems so that he can fit into society successfully.

Some of these identifiable problems exhibited by clients include such factors as self-image and emotional maturity, handling of tensions and frustrations, interpersonal relationships, home and family adjustments, use of leisure time, communication, problems in sexuality, travel, money management, consumer education, and orientation to services within the community. Good physical health is a very basic adjustment problem of enormous importance. Closely related to good physical health are eating habits, personal hygiene, and maintaining a good physical appearance. My previous experience

141

working with the severely disabled as an evaluator at a hospital in Texas showed many clients coming back for medical services over and over again simply because they did not take care of themselves.

Additional crucial adjustment factors include: How do we match the individual's interests, desires and abilities to jobs? How do we teach adequate, work-related concepts of personality and habits needed for competitive or sheltered employment? How do we teach skills needed in finding and interviewing for jobs, as well as skills and training for specific occupations?

These adjustment areas I have mentioned are by no means unique to the severely disabled or handicapped. These problems are universally shared by all human beings. I think we all realize that people are, in fact, more alike than they are different, and to the extent that they do differ, they differ more in degree than in kind. I have a very strong bias against classifying individuals by their categorical disability rather than their functional disability. This is even further compounded by the automatic division between the handicapped and the rest of the human race. The federal government makes the situation even worse by further fragmenting and compartmentalizing the handicapped in the allocation of its money. I remember the big emphasis on the retarded during the Kennedy years, for example. Then came the emphasis on the blind, next the deaf, then the disadvantaged, and now we're on the severely disabled.

I can appreciate that Congress is in a double bind. They are running the largest business operation in the world and are held accountable for investments that should demonstrate commensurate benefits flowing back to the nation. However, political reality dictates that members of Congress respond sensitively to special interest groups among their constituency. The result is a short-range, year-by-year approach to our problems in rehabilitation.

As I have stated, we have in rehabilitation a constantly changing focus, a sort of a Disability-of-the-Year-Plan in which a specific disability receives top billing and the spotlight on center stage. Then, when the year passes, it too is relegated into the shadows backstage. Too often, the important program development and/or insights gained during that year must be prematurely dropped, often just short of reaching the goal. Then everyone in the field surges into the newly designated area of disability because, after all, that is the only area where money is available for the continued operation of his rehabilitation center.

I feel that the interests of both the nation and the handicapped would be better served with a larger scope program that seeks to identify those needs common to all handicapped persons and includes provisions for special delivery systems to meet the need dictated by the nature of the handicap. The goals of such a large scope program would be (1) the development of pragmatic, functionally operative programs and (2) the training of persons in the proper use of those programs in order to guarantee their adequate implementation.

Because Congress and rehabilitation services are pressured to show evidence of increased closures, both are often forced to choose short-range rather than long-term goals. We consistently use the argument that we are saving society money by recycling valuable human resources and making them financially independent.

Available money is already very limited and there is little indication that there will be more. Who will then make the important decisions about how these funds will be used and for whom? With existing funds available, do your priorities dictate placing 200 disadvantaged, or 100 retarded or severely disabled clients, in competitive employment? Unemployment conditions will also affect these figures in placing individuals in competitive employment. If unemployment reaches 8 to 10 percent, can we justify stating that the handicapped need jobs more than individuals who are not handicapped? If the jobs are not available, what happens then to our numbers of successful courses? Who can make, who will make, the decisions about who will be served in order to get the most good for the limited funds available?

When money for any purpose is limited, there is greater societal emphasis on using it for purposes that will show the greatest rate of return on one's investment. A professor on my doctoral committee long ago suggested that using our resources to educate gifted children more adequately would ultimately pay for every retarded program in existence. My response, which has grow in conviction over the years, was "Yes, but the retarded are human beings and need the same chance at life as anyone else." Even in times of plenty there is a strong resistance to the expense of rehabilitation programs. Changes in attitude are more desperately needed now than ever before in order to maintain the financial commitment needed to do the job.

I guess in my idealism that I would like to see programs set up to meet personal individual needs, rather than saying to sequential individuals, "You go to rehab because they cover your classification; you go to Social Security; and you, there, go to Department of Labor projects." Instead, I wish we had one Department of Human Resources that would handle all programs for human needs. This would save money and avoid a tremendous amount of duplication. Then on a systematic basis we would be able to provide more help for all individuals who need it.

Now to get back to the real world. I do feel that working with the severely disabled poses some unique problems that need discussion. The first issue is one of attitude and expectations. The particular factor operating against the resolution of the problems of the severely disabled is often not his adjustment problem per se, nor even his handicap in total, but the attitude with which he and those working with him approach it. This attitude will determine the client's success or failure and whether the diagnosis does in fact become a self-fulfilling prophecy. If your staff has a defeatist attitude toward the retarded, the paraplegic, the quadriplegic—an attitude that says the individual will not make it—I will guarantee that he is not going to make it. This doubt or defeatist attitude is never explicitly expressed to the individual; however, the real message always gets through. The staff members somehow communicate it just as effectively as if they had told it outright.

When dealing with the adjustment problems of the severely handicapped, it is essential that the staff be believers who are committed to giving everything they've got to their work. They must *know* that their clients, aided by the personal and professional support of the staff, are going to make it. The difficult part lies not only in finding staff with these qualities, but in helping them maintain them. The real reward for staff does not come in salaries or desirable working conditions; it comes from helping people. However, change comes very slowly when working with the severely handicapped, and is often frustrating and discouraging. What happens to morale when it takes eight or nine months, or even one or two years, before you can experience a little success?

The attitude that the client must be able to do something is needed to maintain staff morale. Our challenge is to find out what it is. If the client does not have the abilities to be placed in competitive employment, we must not use insight and experience to find other areas in which he can be a contributing member of society. People in the rehabilitation field need the conviction that even though an individual will not be paid a self-sustaining wage, he can succeed at something that gives him a sense of self worth. Staffers need the ingenuity, or at least the tenacity, to hang in there and discover what that something is. You can collect reams of data and develop any number of personal and work adjustment programs for any and every group, however, and still never get off the ground in a successful rehabilitation program. It is the attitude of the individual himself and of those individuals working with him that will make or break any program. Complicating the staff's own personal tendencies to want clients from among the walking wounded with whom they can experience a more gratifying success rate, there is enormous outside pressure as well. Much of it is manifested as financial "incentive" to play the "numbers game." This was mentioned before in reference to the decisions Congress has to make in allocating and justifying funds.

A second concern in working with the severely disabled is that, while they often display a tendency to be extremely dependent, it is our job to strive to make them independent. Their need to maintain that dependency has developed some of the world's most fantastic manipulators: "You wheel me up front," "Start my car." Even though I'm aware of their manipulation, I've been caught in it time and time again. We must allow him the opportunity to learn to do for himself, but, if the client is not motivated to want help in achieving independence, no rehabilitation staff anywhere can be of service to him. The staff must take its frame of reference from the client's perspective. What is it he wants? How does he see himself? The client's own copcept of his problem, unless it is a realistic one, can preclude his ability to cope or achieve his goals. We're handicapped in vocational evaluation when medical doctors, for whatever reason, fail to level with a client or assess for him the possibilities of where he can realistically expect to go with his disability.

An additional concern with the severely disabled is in their attitude toward assistive devices used to lessen their disabilities. Hearing aids, eye glasses, prostheses, and crutches are often found in closets.

We not only have to make our clients functional as possible before evaluation, but we must work with these clients to assist them in accepting and using these devices.

Perhaps I've been repeating myself in stressing the need for experienced staff in working with the severely disabled, but I don't think there is an individual in any program who does not know the importance of good staff. It is the staff who makes the program. To assist the staff in developing adjustment programs for the severely disabled, I'd like to mention some available useful materials. Much of the adjustment material is distributed and developed by the Materials Development Center (MDC). There is a great deal of curriculum material available on adjustment programs. One such manual distributed by the MDC is *Road to New Horizons*, which was developed at Gracewood State Hospital in Georgia. Subtopics include self-evaluation, personal health and hygiene, personal appearance and grooming, basic etiquette, social relationships, use of leisure time, money management and consumer education, home and family adjustment, and community orientation.

The MDC has published as a reprint Gellman's *Adjusting People to Work*. Auburn University has published *Adjustment Services in Rehabilitation* by Baker and Sawyer and does an excellent job in describing the components and considerations for setting up adjustment programs. The MDC, along the same lines, will distribute a sound/slide presentation early in 1975 called *The Work Adjustment Program—An Overview*. As a good example of the cooperation that exists between Stout and Auburn, the MDC also distributes the *Grooming for Men* program, which was developed at Auburn University. By late 1975 the MDC will have a program on *Grooming for Women*.

Since behavior identification is of great importance in adjustment programming, the MDC has published *Observation and Client Evaluation in Workshops*, developed by Chicago JVS, and the *MDC Behavior Identification Format*. Coming soon in 1975 from the MDC will be a selected bibliography on behavior modification and token economies, in addition to sound/slide programs on development of adjustment plans, modeling, token economy as used in rehabilitation programs, and a three-part program in job seeking skills called the *MDC Job Quest Series*.

Comprehensive and potentially excellent audio-visual materials are also available. I say potentially excellent material because its ultimate value is determined by how it is used. If the staff member merely exposes his clients to the film or whatever without first attempting to involve each individual in it at a personal, meaningful level, the material has little value. If, on the other hand, he makes them (1) aware of their own individual needs, (2) builds their desire to overcome those needs, (3) exposes them to material that tells them how, and (4)) subsequently discusses and demonstrates it with them, then and only then does it have potential value.

So again, the staff member is the essential ingredient in the success of a program. The MDC is limited in the effective utilization of its materials because it does not have a training component to teach the most effective use of its materials. We are also impeded by the apathy among many persons in the field in the use of materials. Thus, we are constantly seeking ways of motivating people to get into the material and to implement it. Becoming familiar with what they have right on their resource shelves is absolutely basic. The best information in the world can do no good sitting undiscovered in someone's file cabinet.

Although frustrated and limited by what often happens to material after it leaves us, our commitment continues to be developing materials that will provide assistance to people in the field. Everything we send out is followed up with evaluation forms to determine the material's effectiveness. Over and over again we ask, "What do you want?" "What materials do you need in the field?" I have briefly mentioned only some of the existing MDC materials. Any centers eligible for MDC services can define the areas in which they want material, and the MDC will locate all such material through its information and retrieval system. As things currently stand, it is up to programs like Auburn's and The University of Tennessee's Continuing Education program to provide the training to make our materials usable. We lack our own training component, and their help will be of even greater value than before in the "how-to-do-it" materials the MDC is currently developing.

What I've been saying could be summed up under the single statement that I do not think massively different new programs that again start from the beginning are what can best serve the needs of the very severely disabled. Instead, I'm suggesting that we analyze the needs of individuals, rather than looking at specific handicaps a year at a time. The next step then is to extract from our vast store-houses of professional expertise the delivery systems or adaptations thereof that can implement the programs that will meet those identi-fied needs.

The Fair Labor Standards Act and Wage Payments As Related to the Handicapped in the Tennessee Vocational Training Centers

Latest amendments to the Wage-Hour Law applicable to clients of the Tennessee Vocational Training Centers are discussed. Basic provisions of the Act in relation to employment in workshops are highlighted, restrictive standards and record-keeping requirements are mentioned, and the application of the Walsh-Healy Public Contracts Act is explained.

A work-activity center as part of the workshop is described, as are requirements for meeting one of two productivity tests, requirements for evaluation and/or training programs, and wage rates for these programs.

A question and answer session clarifies many points as to the intent of the law.

In 1938, Congress passed the Fair Labor Standards Act, which is known as the Wage-Hour Law. This act provided for a minimum wage, overtime compensation, child labor provisions, and some other provisions. It has been amended a number of times since then. The latest amendments took effect May 1, 1974. At that time, the state training centers were exempt. They were excluded from the federal law. There was an exclusion in the law for state employees, and we had held that this exclusion would apply to clients of the Tennessee Vocational Training Centers. Therefore, these clients were excluded from the provisions of the Fair Labor Standards Act. Effective May 1, the Fair Labor Standards was amended, and the State Vocational Training Centers are now subject to this law.

The Fair Labor Standards Act fosters job opportunities, however, for those who are unable to earn the minimum wage under the law by authorizing the employment of handicapped workers at special minimum wages that are lower than the statutory minimum wage. At the same time the Act looks out for the monetary interest of the handicapped individual by providing that these special rates may be paid only under certificates that are issued by the Wage-Hour Division and are subject to the conditions that are set forth in the Act and in our regulations, Part 525. (Regulations will be sent upon request by writing to Wage-Hour Division, 1717 West End Building, Room 307, Nashville, Tennessee, 37203.) Other provisions of the Act are applicable to the clients. These include the overtime provisions, the equal pay provisions, and equal pay for equal work regardless of sex.

Questions have been raised concerning staff employees. The staff employees who are handicapped do not qualify for special minimum wages under your Shelter Workshop Certificate. They must be individually certified under a different regulation, Regulation 524. Staff workers are identified in the Regulations, Section 525.11. There you will see that office managers, bookkeepers, and truck drivers are not considered clients. Usually the test for client status is "Does this person serve other clients?" If the answer is yes, then there is usually a staff relationship rather than a client relationship.

Before discussing in more detail the terms and conditions of Shelter Workshop Certificates and the Regulations, I'd like to highlight briefly the basic provisions of the Act in relation to employment in workshops. The Act applies to employees engaged in interstate commerce, or in the production of goods for interstate commerce, and employees of certain enterprises. Enterprise coverage has now been expanded, as I mentioned previously, to include employees of states. Therefore, State Vocational Training Centers are subject. The term "employee" includes persons employed by Shelter Workshops, referred to as clients. Those who are covered, unless specifically exempt, must be paid a minimum wage of $2 an hour. That's the minimum wage at the present time. On January 1, 1975, this will increase to $2.10 an hour. On January 1, 1976, it will increase to $2.30 an hour. These employees must be paid overtime compensation of not less than one and one-half times the regular rate of pay for all hours worked over forty in any work week. Notice the regular rate of pay. This is not time and a half the $2 rate. But if you have a person on your staff who is not exempt, paid $3 an hour we'll say, and he works overtime, he must be paid time and a half at the $3 rate, or $4.50 an hour for the time that is in excess of forty hours in any one particular work week. The employer is required to pay equal pay, regardless of sex, for equal work in jobs that require equal skill, effort, and responsibility and are performed under similar working conditions. Wage differentials are permitted where they are based on a seniority system, merit system, a system which measures earnings by quantity or quality of work, or any factor other than sex.

Under the child labor provision, sixteen years is a minimum age for most employment that is covered by the Act. There is also an eighteen year-old minimum for occupations that have been declared hazardous by the Secretary of Labor. There are some seventeen of these hazardous occupations. In all of the states, there are state child labor laws. On occasion, these laws will differ somewhat from the federal law. If the state has a standard that is more restrictive than the federal standard, you must comply with that standard. If the federal law is more restrictive, then you must comply with that. And it is also true that we don't have a minimum wage law in the state of Tennessee. If any of you should move to another state and there is a minimum wage law there, and if it has higher standards than the federal law, then, as a general rule, you must comply with those standards.

Employers are required to keep records on wages and hours that are worked and other items that are listed in the record-keeping regulations, Part 516. Most of this required information is kept by employers as a matter of ordinary business practice, or in compliance with other laws and regulations. No particular form or order of records is mandatory. There are certain additional record-keeping requirements for certificated Shelter Workshops. These requirements are intended to provide information to substantiate the need for workshop certificates and the adequacy of the wages that are paid. Records of disability, medicals and so forth, must be kept for each client in addition to records that reflect the productivity of each client on a continuing basis for periodic intervals, not to exceed six months. Since relatively few Shelter Workshops perform on government contracts subject to the Walsh-Healey Public Contracts Act, I'll be very brief in my reference to this law, which is also administered by my office. The Act applies to workers who are employed on government supply contracts that are in excess of $10,000 and require payment of the minimum wages that are determined by the Secretary of Labor to be prevailing in that particular industry. These minimums range from $2 an hour. It's at least the minimum wage that is applicable under the Fair Labor Standards Act. At the present time, that would be $2.00. However, in some instances, these wages are higher; it may be $2.50, for example, in a particular industry. When you get a contract of this nature, you'll know. It will be specified in the contract. However, handicapped clients at Shelter Workshops may be employed at lower rates upon the same terms and conditions as prescribed for the employment under Fair Labor Standards Acts and the regulations of 525, the Shelter Workshop regulations. The Public Contract Acts overtime provisions require payment of time for hours over eight hours a day or over forty a week, whichever is greater. There are also requirements concerning safety and health and child labor provisions under that law.

Your workshop may serve multi-handicapped clients who are more or less in complete terminal employment. I don't like the word terminal, but I don't suppose any of you people do any more than I do; I use it only as a means of conveying to you what I mean. I hope you'll never consider any client that you have as a terminal case. However, this very restricted type of client, the multi-handicapped client or the mentally retarded client, is the type that should be in a work activity center. A workshop must meet the definition of a work activity center that is stated in Regulation 525, Section 525.2(c). It must be a separate department of the workshop with separate records and supervision. Here I'm talking about where you also have a regular work program. Certainly, if it were just a work activity center by itself it wouldn't be separated to meet all of this.

You have two productivity tests, and you must meet one of these. The average annual productivity per handicapped client must be less than $1,075. This is a recent increase. Previously this figure was $850. Each of the training centers in Tennessee met this test, the $850 test, because we were testing prior to the time of this increase. There are additional increases in this particular test. This $1,075 figure will increase to $1,125 effective January 1, 1975, and to $1,225 effective January 1, 1976. In order to determine if you meet this test, you would divide the total annual earned income of the work program, less the cost of purchased materials, by the average number of clients in the work programs. In other words, if you had $10,000 gross earned income, $1,000 of that 10,000 might be for materials that you used up; for example, if you were making wood pallets and you bought $1,000 worth of wood to generate this $10,000 income, then you would use the $9,000 figure and divide this by the average number of clients that you had in your work program during that period of time. If this figure were less than $1,075 you would qualify as a work activity center, or, rather, you would meet this test. And I'm assuming that you would meet the other tests that we've already mentioned.

The second test can be used where Wage Payments are primarily at piece rates. "Primarily" means half; i.e., if at least half of your clients are paid piece rates, then you could also have a shot at the second test. If you pay hourly rates, or if over 50 per cent of your clients are paid hourly rates, you must meet the first test. You do not have the opportunity on the second test. On the second test, you take the total annual wages paid to all clients and divide this figure by the average number of clients. This is only the handicapped clients working under this certificate. You do not include staff members. Divide this figure by the average number of clients that you had in the program for that year and, if the result is less than $750 at the present time, then you would qualify under this test. You must meet one of the two tests. The $750 test has recently been increased from $600.

If you qualify for a work activity center certificate there is no specified minimum wage floor. However, clients must be paid a wage that is commensurate with those paid non-handicapped workers in private industry for essentially the same type, quantity and quality of work. We'll talk about this in a minute. I want to go ahead just a few steps further and talk about some other certificates, and then we'll talk about this principle which is applicable for all certificates.

Looking to future certification that you'll have to have in the training centers, you may wish to apply for an evaluation and/or training program. Some shops have only the evaluation program. When we talk about evaluation we're talking about that initial period of time when you are trying to decide what to do with a client, what type of work to place him on. These programs cannot be longer than six months; that is, no client can be in the program for over six months. Of course the program can be renewed as you have a new group of clients come in. You can put these clients in the evaluation program, but no client can be in an evaluation program for longer than six months. During the evaluation period there is no minimum specified. Again, it's similar to the work activity center certificate. However, the commensurate wage rate principle does apply during this period of time.

Following the evaluation period, the client may then be recommended for a training program. Such a program cannot be longer than twelve months except in certain exceptional cases, and in some cases may be less than twelve months, depending on the type of program. For example, a work conditioning program that was not at all involved might require only six months for completion. A printing training program which requires a great deal of skill—and of course we're looking to the type of clients that you are working with—may involve a longer period of time. These training programs must be broken down in certain distinct phases or steps. You must start with Step 1: you list what you plan to teach during that particular step or phase. There must be a related wage rate for each particular step if you are paying hourly rates. In other words, what productive level do you expect of the average client during each step? What do you expect to teach a client in this first phase, and how do you expect him to measure up against non-handicapped employees in private industry during each step? In the first phase you may expect him to do 15 per cent of what a non-handicapped person would do in private industry, and then we want you to pay him 15 per cent of the rate that is prevailing in private industry for that type of work. In Step 2, you may expect him to produce 25 per cent, and so forth. These steps in the training program should be geared so that at the conclusion of the training period the client would then be placed in private industry, if that is your objective, and be paid at least the prevailing wage for that type work.

Question from the floor: You've got a program in a facility that teaches custodial training. The first time that you clean the floor in the place, the facility may be getting a service because you are actually getting a cleanup job. However, what you are actually doing is going back and throwing sawdust or putting gum on the floor because it is strictly training. Are you stating that you have to pay the clients as if they are at 20 per cent of production even though it is training? Since you're making no money or anything out of this, should you be paying the client? *Response:* Yes, sir. If it is the requirement of the law.

Question from the floor: Going one step further. Say you've got a drafting class, but you are working on no contracts, or anything else. You're teaching them how to do drafting. This is a six-month training program. By the same token you should be paying those clients although you are receiving no money? *Response:* If there is no productive work involved, you would not be required to pay them. But if it is productive work . . . .

Question from the floor: How do you define productive work? *Response:* Something that would be of some economic value. If you had an arrangement with an architectural firm where some of the work was sold by the workshop to the architectural firm, then it would be productive work, and you would have to pay them in that case. Normally speaking, they are doing the drawings for their own benefit. When I was in drafting school in the Army, I would roll my drawings all up and store them at home in the attic, which was not of any benefit to anybody.

Question from the floor: This is a facility here and we want them to learn how to clean a rug. The rug is great right now. I come in and I throw sawdust and ashes all over the rug. This is a setup. This is not productive. *Response:* No, it would not be in that particular case. I think your first illustration, though, was going into the plant and doing something there which would be productive work, and this is the type of thing I was speaking of at first. Does everyone understand what we are saying on this? I appreciate your bringing this up, Dr. Sax, because there could be training programs where there would not be productive work, and you are not required under this law to pay clients for that type of work.

Question from the floor: Can I make one more comment? I was talking about the client wage of some of the work activity centers. You should be careful of this because if one of your clients makes too much money it could have a negative effect. In Laredo, Texas, they closed up a workshop under a work activity certificate because clients were making too much money. You've got to watch this. *Response:* Who closed it up? *From the floor:* The Department of Labor. *Response:* That is unfortunate. We've had that occur with a workshop due to the fact that the clients were such high producers that the Work Activities Center was above the annual productivity test and they didn't qualify. Congress has indicated what they meant by work activity centers when they added this to the law in 1966. We certainly don't have the authority to come along and change it to meet the needs of this particular situation here, so we are bound pretty much by what they said. Until they change it, we've got to live with it. I've never closed a workshop and I hope none of you ever feel like I am out there to close down your workshop. I'm not. I guarantee you that I have the same interest that you have in placing handicapped people; that is, to rehabilitate them for work. I'm quite pleased with the regulation that we have. I think if the workshop will comply with the regulations we have with respect to the wage rates, etc., that you'll do an excellent job. I think wages can be an incentive to rehabilitation. I don't think anybody would question that. The regulations have been developed by people like you who have served on the Sheltered Workshop Advisory Committee to the Department of Labor since 1938.

Question from the floor: On the work activity centers that we've got set up in the state funded by VPW, VPW has now come out with a new ruling that they can work half of their working day on contract work. Okay, some of these are in conjunction with places that have shelter workshops that are operating under certificates. Others are not. Are those people applying to you for a special work activity certificate and, if they are not, shouldn't they do it? *Response:* I don't know. I can't say because I don't know who they are, but they should. I've had a few recently and maybe that's why they are being sent in. A lot of times I just have a request, "Please send me the forms necessary to have my program approved." I hope the work is coming down from proper agencies that they must have a certificate before they can pay less. A workshop that does not have a certificate and is doing work covered under the Fair Labor Standards Act must pay all employees, including handicapped clients, at least the minimum wage unless a certificate has been issued that would approve a rate less than the minimum wage. If they are not certified, then they are creating a liability. The difference in what they are paying and $2.00, the minimum wage at this time, may be their liability. If they pay $.10 cents an hour or $.30 cents an hour, they are liable for a difference between that and the $2.00 rate. Just let your imagination go with that and then go over the statutory limitation period of two years, 104 weeks, and you build up a terrific liability. The client has the independent right to sue the workshop for that liability; he can also sue for liquidated damage which can be up to an equal amount. So if you had a $20,000 liability, he could sue for $40,000. I don't say that to scare you, but the individual has the right to do it.

We were talking about training programs. Phase 1 may be for two weeks or whatever. It may just involve safety, just teaching this class how to be safe on the job. Phase 2 may be something involving only hand tools that would be used for this particular occupation, and then Phase 3 may be maintenance of equipment, and so forth. You'd progress, of course; you are building on your program; and each step or phase gets a little bit more skill involved, and the rate should increase.

Assume that you have a client who has completed his evaluation period and he goes into a training program, a work conditioning program of twelve-months duration. At the end of that time he's still in your workshop. You've got to do something else with him. Now, some workshops have a regular work program certificate, and on this type of certificate the minimum floor rate cannot be less than 50 per cent of the minimum, so at the present time this would be $1.00 per hour. When the client completed the evaluation and training program, he would then have to be paid at least $1.00 an hour to stay in this regular work program. In some workshops this is the only type of program, the regular work program. They are not working with clients who are that severely handicapped, so they are able to pay at least 50 per cent of the minimum to all clients. These particular certificates might also occasionally be issued at a rate more than 50 per cent, say $1.25 an hour. You can have a learning period approved that is a low as 50 per cent or $1.00 an hour for a period of time, not to exceed 480 hours. A lot of the Goodwill Shops have this type of program.

In establishing wage rates, if you are paying piece rates and you have a plant manufacturing widgets and in private industry they pay their people $3.00 an hour for the manufacture of these widgets and their normal non-handicapped employee turns out ten of these widgets, that's $.30 cents per unit. So this is what you must pay in the workshop. You must pay $.30 cents per unit in the workshop. You may be paying hourly rates. Sometimes you will have some occupations for which it's almost mandatory that you pay hourly wages. For example, your janitorial people, your maintenance people—you usually can't pay them on a piece rate basis so you must pay them on an hourly basis. You can use a productivity record or a progress report in lieu of a productivity record to establish the hourly rate. Some of the large workshops have maybe ten or fifteen different contracts with that many different piece rates. Seldom will the piece rates be the same. So this presents rather a large task for bookkeepers. I'm thinking about where the client may be moving around on several different piece rates, and if you have 35 or 40 clients and four or five different rates within one week, it's rather difficult to make these calculations.

For that reason, even in a production situation, you may want to pay an hourly rate. This is permissible. You must keep some type of productivity record that would substantiate the adequacy of this particular wage rate that you're paying. These production reports must be kept at intervals not exceeding six months and should be more frequent, depending on the particular set of circumstances that you're operating under. For example, when a client first comes in the program, I think—and I'm not a specialist in this field, and Dr. Sax and Dr. Couch, you correct me if I'm wrong—I think that as a client comes into a workshop program, you'll see that in most cases his production will go almost straight up in those first several months. And then I think, after a period of time, it will begin to level off. The rate of ascent will not be as great after a period of time. In this initial period of time after the client comes in it's going to be necessary for you to make these studies more frequently than you would in the same period of time on down the line after production levels off. We want you to arrive at a wage rate that would be fair. If you have a certificate approved by my office, I'll be sending you a copy of a study, along with a copy of a progress report that has been adopted by the Department of Labor for use for hourly rate clients.

The emphasis on this particular progress report is on quantity and quality of work only. We used to have a form that took into consideration other facts. It took into consideration, for example, attendance, attitude towards other clients, attitude towards supervisors, and things of this nature, which would not be factors to be considered in private industry. However, these studies show that these factors have not reflected a rate that would be commensurate with those paid in private industry. If I may go back, if a client in your workshop turned out six of the units, compared to ten units of normal productivity, normal non-handicapped productivity, prevailing wage rate of $3, the rate must never be lower than the minimum that is applicable, which at the present time is $2. You divide ten into $3.00 giving $.30 cents an hour. If you have a client who is producing say six units, then he would be paid six times $.30 or $1.80 an hour.

Several years ago, in bidding contracts, we required that you have at least 100 per cent overhead of the labor cost. So if you found $.30 cents a unit for your labor cost—your direct labor cost—we wanted you to bid another $.30 cents for your overhead. I don't know whether you've done this in your timing centers or not. If you took the accounting records of the average manufacturing plant, you would find that the overhead was 100 per cent of the direct labor costs of a particular product. So that's why we used the 100 per cent overhead. If you're not charging the employer with this overhead, then to my way of thinking you are subsidizing his business. Whether we require it or not, I think it is really unwise for a workshop to take a contract for only the direct labor. We can't do anything about it even if you take it for less, but you must pay the per unit direct labor cost to your client. So, if you bid anything less, you're going to have to subsidize it yourself out of some fund. If you bid anything more, you don't have to pay it to the client. You can keep this to defray your own overhead costs. It won't be sufficient to defray the total overhead cost that you have, but you can do that.

If you don't want to do that in the state shops, if your salaries and so forth are paid from state funds and you don't have to worry about that overhead, and you get extra when you go out and bid your contract, you can always come back and give it to the clients. I don't think there is anything wrong with that. I think it would be good if you can. Give them a bonus or something of this nature. I think there may be some merit, although I've had some people question me about it in the past. What if we pay a client and he's worth say $.50 cents an hour and we get this overhead and we pay him $1.00 an hour? Then it comes time to place him in private industry and we can't place him at $1.00 an hour, and the only way we can place him is at $.80 cents an hour, or some lower rate. I think you'll find that private industry will be more willing to subsidize him because they've got, in some of these large plants, thirty-five to forty people or maybe even two or three hundred, depending on the plant, and they can subsidize that rate a whole lot easier than you can in the workshop. So this might not be a problem at all. If you want to do it some other way you might do it by paying him what he would be worth at that particular time and then sit down at the end of the year and give him some type of bonus, or something of this nature, not in the form of a wage.

Question from the floor: This could be a problem, if you are giving clients extra money. What you are trying to get is a realistic picture of how that client produces. I would rather see that money used to provide better service, hire extra staff, take them out to a ball game. *Response:* This is a good point. I was trying to give the other side of the argument that has been used, and I've been challenged on this. It's not a realistic situation when you are paying him more than he's actually producing. This may be the case and it may be better, as you suggested, not to give it to him at that time but to give him a bonus—I'm not sure about the ball game idea. I went to the Atlanta Braves ball game last week. I enjoyed it, but whether my wife enjoyed it, I don't know. I don't think she did really. I think if you could get this fund that you have gotten in overhead back to the client in some way, in some manner other than a wage, or so that he would not think of it in terms of a wage, then you might be a little bit better off.

I want to close by saying that I appreciate what you've done in the past year. I noticed in the paper last night that Mr. Reece is quoted as saying that 7,500 persons had been rehabilitated for work in the State of Tennessee this past year. I would think a lion's share of the credit would go to you people in this room who work in the training centers. I compliment you for your efforts and appreciate what you've done in the past. I look forward to working with you more in the future than I have in the past, and I hope that you will consider me a friend and not consider me as the old fellow in Nashville who is going to whack your hand. I want to work with you in any way we can.

Let me say this about placing clients—I failed to mention this and I think it's important. I think most of you are aware of the fact that clients can be placed in private industry at less than the minimum wage, and I think that perhaps you will find more of this in the future as you try to go out in private industry and place clients at the increased minimum wage of $2.00 an hour, especially out in the rural areas. If you are trying to place a client with a particular factory, you may have to place him at a rate less than the minimum wage. Certificates can be approved for these special rates. Rehabilitation counselors can issue them at 50 per cent of the minimum wage on temporary certificates for ninety days. These must be approved by your regional directors. You know what rate is fair for the client, and I think you know the obligation that you have to him. I don't think you would want to be placed at a rate that was not fair to you, so if you don't think the rate is fair, don't place him there. But if you think it is fair and if you think this presents a good opportunity for the particular individual, place him there even if you have to use a certificate. Send the certificate to your regional director for his approval and send a copy to me. This is a temporary certificate now, for ninety days, and then it can be extended if necessary, indefinitely, as a matter of fact. It would have to be renewed periodically.

Harold W. Haddle, Jr.

Behavior Change Through Self-Control
A Training Model for Helping the Severely Disabled

Various approaches to self-control training are presented in this paper as alternatives or adjuncts to traditional insight-oriented psychotherapy for assisting severely disabled persons with psychological problems. Anxiety-reduction training is a useful approach for the rehabilitation counselor to use with clients who experience maladaptive anxiety. Assertive training is a useful approach for helping clients to cope verbally with interpersonal difficulties and to learn social skills.

Perhaps the most difficult question a rehabilitation counselor must face when working with severely disabled clients with psychological problems is, "What behavior change approach works best?" As a former rehabilitation counselor working with clients who lacked social skills and had long histories of chronic psychological malfunctioning, this writer found severe limitations in the exclusive use of insight-oriented psychotherapy to produce significant functional change. It has also been demonstrated that traditional approaches fail for "lower and working class" patients since a more problem-solving, active involvement on the part of the counselor is expected by these groups (Goldstein, 1973). When a counselor is limited to the use of one approach, it is apparent that the scope of his or her effectiveness will be limited.

To meet the psychological needs of a severely disabled population, it seems necessary for the rehabilitation counselor to equip himself with as many helping skills as possible. The purpose of this article is to discuss the use of two "self-control" training techniques to assist clients in improving their psychological function. "Self-control" training, as used in this paper, involves the client's active involvement in planning and implementing behavioral change programs for himself.

161

RATIONALE FOR SELF-CONTROL TRAINING

"'Self-control" training probably has its roots in Skinner's *Science and Human Behavior* (1953), which is a systematic study of self-modification. In his book, he listed eight ways of achieving self-control. Others have elaborated on self-control training strategies, linking these to a general theory of behavior (Ferster, 1965; Goldiamond, 1965). A practical application of self-control strategies, with self-modification procedures for the layman, has been developed by Watson and Tharp (1972).

The area of attitude change theory and research offers a rationale for self-control procedures. Attitude theorists generally consider attitudes acquisition and change contingent on three major components: affective, behavioral, and cognitive. Various psychotherapeutic and counseling approaches tend to focus primarily on one of these components. For example, counterconditioning techniques, such as systematic desensitization, were originally conceptualized as focusing on the affective, or "feeling" component. Operant conditioning procedures, such as token economics, focused on the behavioral component, while cognitive restructuring procedures such as Ellis' "Rational Emotive Therapy" have focused on the cognitive or "thinking" aspect of attitude.

Recent research and theories in behavior therapy have shown that all of these therapeutic techniques involve teaching patients *self-control*, since not only does a particular method of treatment influence a specific component of attitude, but there is also a "mediating" component which somehow consolidates the various components into a total "gestalt." This "mediating" effect is considered by Goldfried (1972) as evidence that therapeutic techniques can be considered as "training in self-control." He shows, with strong research evidence, specifically how systematic desensitization is not merely a deconditioning procedure which affects the autonomic nervous system while the patient passively receives the treatment, but is rather a process whereby the patient actively learns self-control. He indicates that this active process is "'directed toward learning of a general anxiety-reducing skill rather than the passive desensitization to specific aversive stimuli (p. 288).'"

When one scrutinizes Goldfried's work and Goldstein's (1973), who considers psychotherapy primarily as *training*, it can be concluded that a training paradigm, with the purpose of shaping coping skills through teaching self-control procedures, is a viable alternative to a traditional therapy model.

There are many approaches to "self-control" training. The two areas which this article will focus on are *anxiety reduction training* and *assertive training*.

ANXIETY REDUCTION TRAINING

Anxiety is an important construct when analyzing human behavior. We could not function without experiencing some level of anxiety. We encounter difficulties, however, when anxiety becomes unmanageable or "maladaptive." Figure 1 (see Appendix C) illustrates a contrast of individual functioning between one who is managing his anxiety (adaptive))and one who is not managing his anxiety (maladaptive). The adaptive pattern is one of (1) psychological openness to one's environment, and (2) good contact with reality. In contrast, the maladaptive patterns involves (1) a lack of psychological openness and (2) a distorted view of reality, which are determined by an unmanageable level of anxiety. It is interesting to note that the "neuroses," as described by DSMII, are characterized chiefly by anxiety. Psychotic disturbances, likewise, are exacerbated by inappropriate management of anxiety.

Assessment of Anxiety Level

In assisting persons to develop self-control procedures to reduce maladaptive anxiety, it is helpful to teach them ways to assess their level of anxiety. One way to do this is illustrated in Chart 1 (see Appendix C). The "Anxiety Indicator Chart" can teach one to assess his anxiety level by becoming aware of his feelings as they relate to his mental and physical state. The measure of anxiety is categorized according to various activity levels within the brain (delta, theta, alpha, and beta). In practice, one learns to view his anxiety level as if looking at an imaginary "anxiety thermometer" (see Chart I). With some practice, clients can learn to assess with generally good accuracy their anxiety "temperature."

Relaxation Training

Relaxation training can be initiated with clients who suffer from maladaptive anxiety. This is a skill which can be taught individually or within a group setting. First, the client should be taught how to assess anxiety level; then, relaxation training can be initiated.

The most common form of relaxation training is deep muscle relaxation. In selecting physically disabled clients for relaxation training, however, the counselor should be sure that none of the exercises exacerbate any existing physical problems. If clients are severely physically disabled (quadraplegia, rheumatoid arthritis, etc.) a form of relaxation training using suggestion rather than deep muscle relaxation is recomended. (For suggestion techniques, see Zaffuto, 1974; Benson, 1975).

A procedure for learning to teach the skill of relaxation training is simple, which is a primary reason for utilizing this approach to begin self-control training. A basic exercise for deep muscle relaxation can be found in Appendix C. The counselor should begin to do relaxation training by learning how to effectively use the various approaches on himself. A good place to start is to record the relaxation instructions in Appendix C on a cassette tape. Play the tape over and over until you are able to reach, by your own assessment, the alpha level, as found in Chart I. Then, try the instructions with a friend or colleague until you can successfully help him to relax, or reach the alpha level of activity. After you have successfully completed these activities, you should be ready to help your clients to assess anxiety and to teach them deep muscle relaxation.

It is probably best to instruct clients to relax on an individual basis, initially, making "homework" assignments to insure that self-management progresses. Give a copy of your tape to your client (or have him make his own) to use, preferably, twice daily, and have bi-weekly sessions (30 minutes is usually sufficient) for the first couple of weeks. These sessions can be used for clients to practice relaxation and for feedback about their progress in self-management.

After you have relaxed individuals, you should be ready to set up a relaxation training group to teach clients how to manage maladaptive anxiety. A very helpful format for presenting the rationale for a relaxation training group is given by Dr. Arnold Lazarus in a cassette tape, "Use of Relaxation," a part of series entitled, "Daily Living: Coping with Tensions and Anxieties" (IDI, 1970).

Cognitive Restructing for Anxiety Relief Training

Albert Ellis stresses that a human being "can be rewarded or punished by his own thinking . . ." (1962, p. 16). Shakespeare cited in Hamlet, "There is nothing either good or bad but thinking makes it so." How we perceive situations contributes significantly to how we respond behaviorally. Cognitive restructing approaches faciliate clients in thinking differently about situations.

Anxiety as a maladaptive behavior can be triggered by our thinking illogical thoughts. As a part of anxiety-relief training it can be helpful to clients to learn, as self-control skills, cognitive restructing approaches to manage maladaptive anxiety.

Thought Stopping

Several cognitive restructing approaches to manage anxiety are cited by Lazarus (1971). One of these approaches is the "thought-stopping" technique. Basically, the counselor teaches the client how to control obsessive anxiety-provoking thoughts through covert self-talk. A procedure for teaching clients this approach is as follows:

The counselor instructs the client to begin discussing vocally the thought he wishes to control. As the client discusses the thought, the counselor yells, "Stop!" The counselor then asks the client to continue ruminating vocally about other irrational thoughts which are producing anxiety. As soon as these thoughts are elicited, the counselor continues to yell, "Stop!"

The client is then instructed to yell, "Stop!" vocally (overtly) as soon as he elicits vocally his obsessions. The next step involves instructing the client to sub-vocally, or covertly, yell, "Stop!" as he covertly thinks the irrational thoughts. The client then practices this step in the counselor's presence.

After the counselor is confident that the client has learned how to utilize thought-stopping, he assigns the client the task of practicing the technique when irrational thoughts occur. To maximize the self-control aspect, clients should be instructed to keep a diary of when these thoughts occur and the number of times thoughtstopping is applied to each thought. Fensterheim (1975) reports that one of his clients who was using this approach to control "put-down" thoughts used "Stop!" 432 times in a single day. By the end of a week, he was down to only 20 a day.

Two rules which are important to promote success using thought stopping are (Fensterheim, 1975):

1. The client should be taught to use the "Stop!" routine as soon as he is aware of a thought he wants to control.

2. The "'Stop!" routine should be used *every time* the thought occurs.. If not, one may place himself on an intermittent random reinforcement schedule which makes the habit even stronger. It should be used all the time or not at all.

The "Relaxation Response"

Herbert Benson, in his current best-seller, *The Relaxation Response*, presents a simple technique for training patients at Beth Israel Hospital of Boston to reduce anxiety. This approach, which was developed at Harvard's Thorndike Memorial Laboratory, was found to produce the same physiologic changes observed through his group's research on Transcendental Meditation. The technique is being used to lower blood pressure and relieve anxiety in certain hospitalized patients.

In summary, the technique involves (1) getting into a quiet environment, (2) developing a "mental device" (a sound ,word, or phrase repeated silently or aloud, or fixed gazing at an object), (3) developing a "passive" attitude, and (4) maintaining a comfortable position.

Details about the "Relaxation Response" procedure can be found in Benson's book. Basically, the client is instructed to sit quietly, with eyes closed. Relaxation is begun with careful attention paid to breathing. A key word is repeated. A passive attitude is encouraged. This procedure is done from 10 to 20 minutes, once or twice a day.

It is interesting that much of Benson's work as well as the biofeedback research have emphasized the psychophysiologic changes which can occur with the use of various self-control procedures. Then potential use of these approaches with the severely disabled client who has physical and/or emotional problems is encouraging.

Time Projection

The time projection technique (Lazarus, 1971) can reduce anxiety or depression by having the client to imagine himself as being a few days to several years into the future. The counselor teaches the client to imagine himself functioning happily and effectively at that future date. Lazarus (1971) cites an example of a young man who lacked confidence in social situations. He was instructed to picture himself three months into the future where he would be filled with confidence while handling this social situation in mastery. In-between sessions, he was instructed to practice positive imagery several times a day. He gained rapidly in social confidence and skill. His friends and acquaintances confirmed his newfound sense of self-assurance. This procedure also works well with problems of depression since "depression may be regarded as a function of inadequate or unsufficient reinforcers . . . once the patient can imagine himself sufficiently freed from his oppressive inertia to engage in some enjoyable (or formerly enjoyable) activity, a lifting of depressive affect is often apparent (Lazarus, 1968)."

Gendlin's "Focusing" Technique

Gendlin (1969) described an affect-eliciting technique which relies on the client's introspective experience. The client is quietly relaxed and asked to pay attention to his feelings and thoughts until he focuses fully on one special feeling. He "follows" this feeling intensively for a few minutes and then at the end the client is asked to "take what is fresh, or new, in the feel of it now . . . and go very easy." He also is asked to, "Let the words or pictures change until they feel just right in capturing your feelings." The technique shifts the emphasis from superficial thinking and talking about feelings to the actual experiencing of the feelings through bodily expressions. The result of this exercise is often anxiety reduction due to the cathartic and desensitizing nature of the experience.

ASSERTIVE TRAINING

Assertive training is an exceptionally useful approach for helping clients to learn to cope verbally with interpersonal difficulties and to learn social skills. Webster's definition of "assert" is "to state or affirm positively, assuredly, plainly, and strongly." Assertive behavior, according to Alberti and Emmons (1974) is . . . "behavior which enables a person to act in his own best interests, to stand up for himself without undue anxiety, to express his honest feelings comfortably, or to exercise his own rights without denying the rights of others (p. 2)." Improvement of interpersonal skills is a major goal in teaching clients how to cope. Inherent in teaching assertive skills is the philosophy that individuals have basic rights and they can learn to exercise these rights through establishing a behavioral repertoire of verbal coping skills.

According to Fensterheim (1975), and earlier, Salter (1949), "neurotic" problems occur as a result of inappropriate behavior. An inappropriate behavioral response ca ntrigger deprecatory feelings, anxiety, and depression. Assertive training teaches more adequate behavioral responses which should relieve much of the tension and depression resulting from the helpless feeling that one has no control over his own behavior or environment.

There are important distinctions between assertive behavior and two ineffective behavior styles, which may be called non-assertive behavior and aggressive behavior. The person who typically responds in a non-assertive manner is inhibited, self-denying, and likely does not accomplish the goals he sets for himself. He is usually quite dependent on other persons to the extent that he evokes anger or guilt from persons due to his extreme passivity.

Aggressive behavior is an extreme attempt at self-assertion. One who engages in aggressive behavior tends to "put down" and depreciate others. When he gets what he wants, he does so at the expense of others. Extreme examples of aggressive behavior are found in various criminal acts. Less severe aggressive behavior may involve the use of verbally abusive statements to attack another person.

Assertive behavior, in contrast, involves utilizing verbal problem-solving skills in effective self-expression. When one learns to be assertive, he learns that he can control his own behavior and be responsible for it. He exercises the right to choose. Even though there is no guarantee that he will reach his goals, he learns to feel confident about himself because he exercises self-control and learns to avoid being manipulated by other persons.

Teaching Assertive Skills to Severely Disabled Clients

There are broad applications of assertive training for the severely disabled. The psychological problems related to the disability itself and being stigmatized by society can cause feelings of low self-esteem and helplessness on the part of the disabled. Coping in a competitive job market is often a difficulty for the severely disabled person. Applications of assertive training can be made in the following areas:

Job Interviewing
Interpersonal relationships with family and friends

Teaching basic social conversation skills
Coping with bureaucracies
Overcoming depression and anxiety

Assertive Training Groups

In this writer's experience, the use of assertive training groups can be very beneficial for severely disabled persons. Most clients can profit from this training approach and can learn to use assertive training as a self-control procedure. The groups typically meet once a week (1½ hrs.) for 24 weeks. Ideally, the group should consist of 8-10 members.

The following elements have been useful in training chronically disabled psychiatric patients and should be applicable to other disability groups.

Data Collection and Targets of Change

A pre-training interview with a prospective group member to orient the member to the group and to discover the relative priority of problems is highly recommended. It is sometimes helpful to administer an assertiveness inventory. An inventory which this writer has found useful can be found in Alberti and Emmon's *Your Perfect Right.*

It is helpful to teach clients as early as possible in the group to observe their own behavior. This can be done by their keeping a diary of their responses in situations when they were or were not assertive. This approach facilitates clients in determining areas of change they wish to focus on. The next step involves delineating target behaviors to work on, using the self-observations as baseline estimates of the frequency of the problem behaviors. Treatment plans are then developed for each client.

Training Procedures

Major training procedures used in assertive training groups are modeling, coaching, behavior rehearsal, and covert rehearsal.

Modeling is a demonstration of desirable responses to specific problem situations. A modeling tape, which illustrates several assertive responses, is helpful in teaching clients a repertoire of basic skills along with concentrating on individual problems. This writer has developed an audio training tape which models, through role-playing, the differences between assertive, non-assertive, and aggressive behaviors. For practice, group members are later asked to make up their own assertive responses to increasingly difficult situations.

Manuel Smith's (1975) seven "systematic assertive skills" are taught to group members through use of an audio modeling tape and group practice. Sometimes the group is separated into dyads to practice the various responses while the leader mills around to offer feedback.

Coaching is a useful procedure in teaching assertive skills. The leader and knowledgeable members are helpful to less knowledgeable members by describing appropriate responses to problem situations and by assisting them to make these responses in the group.

Behavior rehearsal is a major procedure that involves clients in role-playing the skills each is trying to learn.

Covert rehearsal is similiar to behavior rehearsal, except that the client sub-vocally imagines how he would respond in given situations rather than acting or vocalizing in the situation. Clients covertly imagine themselves as effectively dealing with situations, using the assertive style which is "natural" for them. This procedure is practiced and discussed before the actual behavior rehearsal, or role-playing, is enacted in the group.

Group Attractiveness

It is important for the group leader to structure the assertive groups for meaningful interaction to occur. If interaction is too prescribed, the group's attractiveness for members may be limited. To stimulate group attraction, the leader should choose the more difficult situations to role-play during the sessions. Dividing the group into dyads for interviewing and self-disclosure is a way for members to get well acquainted. Encouragement for everyone to speak is essential.

Use of Homework

In assertive training groups, clients are given behavioral assignments to try out between sessions. This aspect of the training is quite important since it focuses on the self-control element of the training. Behavioral assignments also provide material for clients to bring to the group next session for feedback and further work on problem areas.

References

Alberti, R., and Emmons, M. *Your Perfect Right.* San Luis Obispo: IM-PACT Press, 1974.

American Psychiatric Association. *DSMII-Diagnostic and Statistical Manual of Mental Disorders* (Second Edition) Washington, D.C., 1968.

Ellis, A. *Reason and Emotion in Psychotherapy.* New York: Lyle Stuart, 1962.

Fensterheim, H., and Baer, J. *Don't Say Yes When You Want to Say No.* New York: McKay, 1975.

Ferster, C. B. Classification of behavioral pathology. In L. Krasner and L. P. Ullmann (Eds.) *Research in Behavior Modification.* New York: Holt, Rinehart and Winston, 1965.

Gendlin, E. T. Focusing. *Psychotherapy: Theory, Research and Practice,* 1969, 6, 4-15.

Goldiamond, I. "Self-control procedures in personal behavior problems." *Psychological Reports,* 1965, 17, 851-868.

Goldstein, A. *Structured Learning Therapy: Toward a Psychotherapy for the Poor.* New York: Academic Press, 1973.

Instructional Dynamics, Incorporated. *Daily Living: Coping with Tensions and Anxieties.* Chicago, 1970.

Lazarus, A. A. Learning theory and the treatment of depression. *Behavior Research and Therapy,* 1968, 6, 83-89.

Lazarus, A. *Behavior Therapy and Beyond.* New York: McGraw-Hill, 1971.

Salter, A. *Conditioned Reflex Therapy.* New York: Famar, Strauss, 1949.

Skinner, B. F. *Science and Human Behavior.* New York: Macmillan, 1953.

Smith, M. *When I Say No, I Feel Guilty.* New York: Dial Press, 1975.

Watson, D. and Tharp, R. *Self Directed Behavior.* Monterey: Brooks-Cole Publishing Co.

Zaffuto, A. *Alphagenics: How to Use Your Brain Waves to Improve Your Life.* New York: Doubleday, 1974.

Robert E. Tooms

Medical and Psychosocial Problems
of the Spinal Cord Injured Client[1]

The implications of injury to the spinal cord at various sites are presented. Neurological evaluation (including sensory evaluation, muscle testing, and reflex changes) determines the level of the lesion and whether it is complete or incomplete.

Emphasized is the importance of proper emergency care at the time of the injury and the necessity of getting the patient into treatment at a specialized spinal injury center as soon as possible. SCI patients require extremely specialized, very knowledgeable care through a multi-disciplinary team effort. Delay in providing this may cause totally needless complications.

Requirements for optimal rehabilitation of the SCI client, after physical rehabilitation has been accomplished, include vocational evaluation, retraining, and elimination of architectural and transportation barriers. Spinal injury centers must assume the obligation for educating both professional and lay people, as well as patients and their families, regarding these needs.

Ladies and gentlemen, I would like to recognize some of the dignitaries in the audience, but I am afraid to start because I'm sure I'll miss recognizing someone. We certainly have an extremely impressive array of people here in addition to having the vast majority of vocational rehabilitation counselors in the state of Tennessee. We are very flattered and very honored at the opportunity of coming to speak with you today, hopefully to enlighten some of you and to increase the information some of the rest of you already have about what is being done locally in the way of care for the spinal cord injured patient. I see many faces out in the audience that I know. There are many others that I don't know. I am glad to see that some of the vocational rehabilitation counselors are much prettier than some of the ones with whom I'm accustomed to work. Others I have seen before and I am glad to see them again.

Let me try to set the stage for what we are going to talk about today. I want to give you a brief overview of what a spinal cord

173

injury is, how we as physicians attempt to evaluate these people, and then introduce you to the concept of a spinal cord injury center as we see it. I will then introduce to you the various members of the multi-disciplinary group at our own Spinal Cord Injury Center and let them tell you what it is that they, as chiefs of their departments, attempt to do for the spinal cord injured patient. Let me first remind you that spinal cord injury is probably as devastating a physical impairment as one can have. Those of use who deal day in and day out with the spinal cord injured patient are not as impressed with the hopelessness of this situation as perhaps some of you are. We feel that the vast majority of these people are rehabilitatable in the broad sense of the word, and that is why our unit came into being. The Spinal Cord Injury Center at the Lamar Unit of the Baptist Hospital in Memphis was established about five years ago with twenty-three beds for what I refer to as a Phase 2 rehabilitation effort for spinal cord injured patients. (I'll define these phases later). The Lamar Unit of the Baptist Hospital is strictly a rehabilitation hospital and has a total capacity of 125 beds. Therefore, the Spinal Cord Injury Center represents only a small segment of what goes on in the form of rehabilitative efforts in the Lamar Unit.

Now if we could have the lights off and the first slide please, I'd like to acquaint you with a little bit of what we're talking about in rehabilitating the spinal cord injured. This first slide is simply a sagittal section of an injured spinal cord. The bony part that you see represents the vertebral column, and you can see that one vertebra has been shoved forward over another. In the center of the slide there runs a white structure which is the human spinal cord. This human spinal cord is of a toothpaste consistency and is very easily damaged. Once damaged, it does not have the power of regeneration, so, when you see an injury of this sort to the spinal cord, it means that the person who has this particular injury is going to have a complete spinal cord injury for the rest of his life because it is irreversible by any means of which we are now cognizant. Almost 5,000 years ago, a writer wrote into an Egyptian papyrus, the Edwin Smith Papyrus, that a spinal cord injury was "an ailment not to be treated." Unfortunately, this is the attitude that prevailed world-wide until at least the mid-portion of this century. In 1944, toward the end of the Second World War, the spinal cord injury unit at Stoke-Mandeville Hospital in England was established for the care of servicemen who had sustained spinal cord injuries. This, I think, was probably the beginning of the modern approach to the care of patients with spinal cord injuries.

There are a number of factors that influence what we can anticipate in the way of functional return and which also influence our treatment program for patients who have spinal cord injuries. The first of these is called "the level of injury." By this we mean, "Where is the site of the spinal cord injury?" For example, if the spinal cord is injured in the neck, it's a cervical injury. We also like to detail it a bit more and say it's a certain level in the cervical spine such as C-5, C-6, or C-7. All of these things are important to us in localizing the level of injury and are part of the language we speak to each other.

The next thing that I would like to show you is simply the appearance of a human whose skin has been removed and whose spinal cord you can see. All the bony elements have been taken off the back of the vertebral column, and you can see that the spinal cord runs up and down in the middle of the back with the nerve roots coming out to each side. We find that the spinal cord does not run all the way from the skull to the tip of the vertebral column. In fact, it ends at the bottom of L-1 or the top of L-2, which means that some of the segments of the spinal cord become crowded together as one goes from the brain to the tip of the spinal cord. Therefore, spinal cord segmental levels do not correspond with vertebral levels. In clinical practice this means that someone who has a fracture dislocation of T-12 on L-1 doesn't have a neurological level at T-12 or at L-1, but it is actually going to be considerably lower. We also see that somewhere at the bottom of L-1 or at the top of L-2 the spinal cord ends and beyond that all we have are nerve roots. Nerve roots are in essence the same thing as peripheral nerves, and they do have the power of regeneration. An injury in this area is totally different from one of the spinal cord itself, which does not have the power of regeneration.

Now, how do we determine whether or not this spinal cord injury that we're talking about is complete or incomplete, and how do we determine the level of the injury? Of course, we have x-ray studies that will tell us where a bone or vertebral injury is, but where is it as far as the spinal cord is concerned? Is it complete or is it incomplete? We determine this by performing a neurological examination. First of all we do a sensory examination. The human body is very well demarcated as to levels of sensation, and this picture, drawn by Dr. Frank Netter, shows the levels of various sensory dermatomes as you see them numbered. We do a sensory examination to tell us what's functioning and what's not. Where do you lose feeling? Where are you numb? Below what level? This gives us an idea of the level of the lesion. Number two, we do a muscle test, and both the physical and the occupational therapists will be talking to you a bit more about this. Certain muscles receive their nerve supply from certain levels of the spinal cord. If these muscles are paralyzed, then the part of the spinal cord that is the site of origin for those nerves has been damaged, and therefore that muscle is not functioning. This gives us another indication of the level of the injury. We also test the deep tendon reflexes. On all the old movies on TV at nights you'll see the psychiatrist hitting the patients in the knee. That really is not a test to see if you're crazy. It's a part of the neurological examination that lets us know again what level or function has been disturbed. So we use sensory evaluation, muscle testing, and reflex changes, among other things, to tell us what is the level of the lesion and if it is complete or not complete. By being complete, we mean there is no function distal to the level of the lesion. By being incomplete we mean there is some sparing of nerve tissue in the cord so that some function is going through that injured level, and therefore you have some preservation of sensation and some preservation of motor function. This is what we mean by complete or incomplete. An incomplete lesion has the potential for recovering function. A complete lesion, we believe, is essentially going to remain unchanged. You may pick up one or more nerve roots at the level of the lesion. But if there is a complete severance of the spinal cord by a missile, a knife wound, by crushing from a fracture, or dislocation or any other means, then this patient is not going to have a return of function of more than one or two nerve roots from the level of the lesion.

There has been a big hue and cry about whether or not to do a laminectomy on these patients, but I don't think that question concerns this particular audience. We feel there are certain very, very narrow indications for doing a laminectomy, but, in general, most patients don't need it. My neurosurgeon colleagues would probably disagree with the statement, but, again, that is a discussion I think is somewhat inappropriate for this group.

The main thing I want to emphasize this afternoon is the necessity for taking care of people with spinal cord injuries in a specialized center. Over the years those people who have dealt with spinal cord injured patients have found that patients fare much better when they are taken care of by a multi-disciplinary team effort than they do when taken care of in a small community hospital. It's not to say that the doctor or the nurse or the therapist in that small community hospital isn't just as capable as I am or as my nurse or my therapist is, but spinal cord injured patients require extremely specialized, very knowledgeable care, and this type of care is by far and away best rendered in very specialized centers.

The estimate about the incidence of spinal injured patients is that each year somewhere between fifteen and fifty people per million sustain spinal cord injuries. We feel like a good average of this is about thirty. For every million people in the United States, thirty of those people are going to sustain a spinal cord injury in some form or another. That is a relatively small group of people. Probably in the United States at the present time there are some 10,000 to 12,000 people each year who sustain spinal cord injuries. How many of them are here in Tennessee, I honestly don't know. I do know that the state of Arkansas is performing a survey to find out how many spinal cord injured patients live in that state. I think that will be a very interesting statistic, and I'd like to have the same sort of survey done in Tennessee. It would give us a better idea of the magnitude of our problem.

Another thing I want to mention to you is that the care of the spinal cord injured patient doesn't begin when that patient gets to the rehabilitation center, or at least it should not begin then. The spinal cord injured deserves an entire systemic approach. By that I mean you should begin the care of that patient from the time the injury occurs out on the highway, at the swimming pool, or in a nightclub where he's been shot or stabbed; that is, when he is being picked up by the ambulance driver. This means that we must first of all have a good system of emergency evacuation of these people, including both ground transportation and air transportation if necessary. That in turn implies that the people who are going to evacuate these patients must have a certain level of training in order to do this properly and not increase the damage that has already been wrought by the injuries. The next thing it implies is that there must be good communication, hopefully two-way radio communication, between the emergency evacuation unit at the scene of the accident and the hospital emergency room preparing to recive this person. The hospital that is going to receive this patient must be well equipped and also staffed by people who know how to handle this type of patient. They must have proper x-ray equipment and operating rooms as well as surgeons who know how to handle these patients. I think these patients are best treated in an acute injury center. We don't have an acute center, but we're working toward one. We see too many patients who have come to us either two weeks, two months or two years after their injury, who have already developed totally needless complications in the form of pressure sores, flexion contractures, bladder stones, chronic infections, and, perhaps even more important than any of these physical ailments, total psychologic devastation. None of these things is necessary and most can be prevented. Some of them can be prevented completely. For example, pressure sores need never occur. Pressure causes pressure sores and we know how to eliminate pressure. If we get the patients early we can prevent pressure sores. It has been estimated in the past that it costs $5,000 for every single pressure sore a patient gets. Those are old statistics. I think it costs $7,500 for every pressure sore, and we constantly see patients who have two, three, and four pressure sores. This increases the cost to someone of care for that patient: either Tennessee Vocational Rehabilitation, some other governmental agency, or private insurance carrier, and ultimately you and me. In any event, we need to have better established acute centers for the care of these people and rapid transfer to a specialized Phase Two unit like our Spinal Cord Injury Center. Based on government statistics, we should have seventy-five regional spinal cord injury centers in the United States; we probably have about ten. This gives you some idea of the gap between what we should have and what we do have.

Subsequent to the patient's physical rehabilitation, he needs to be evaluated by specialists such as yourselves about whether or not he needs further formal education or further vocational education. That is to say, he needs to have vocational evaluation and retraining. Most of the vocational evaluation and training centers presently in existence are not geared to the very severely disabled patients. They are geared to the less severely disabled patients, and spinal cord injury patients require a different type of setting for evaluation and training. Hopefully in Tennessee we're making good strides towards the establishment of vocational re-evaluation and training centers for the very severely disabled and physically impaired.

Subsequent to the patient's rehabilitation, both physically and vocationally, he has to live somewhere. He has to have transportation back and forth from work. He must have some means for enjoying avocational pursuits. This means the elimination of architectural barriers; this means specialized housing; this means specialized transportation. All of these systems are sorely lacking and we are frustrated by this day in and day out. It does us very little good to completely rehabilitate our patient, teach him maximum independence, and send him from our unit where things are reasonably clean and shiny and nice back to a house without any plumbing inside and where he can't get his wheelchair in or out because it's got ten steps. I'm painting a bad picture of it because I'm trying to bring to your consciousness exactly what some of our problems are.

One of the many obligations that we in spinal injury centers must assume is the education of groups like this—physicians, nurses, therapists, and other people who are participants in the care of these people and for whom there is little offered in the way of educational facilities. We try to do this in our unit. We have students with us in nursing, PT and OT. We also have medical students work with us. There is not only need to educate professional medical people, but there is also a need to educate the general population, the patient, and the patient's family.

Finally, there is the need for research into spinal cord injuries. Why do we have them? How can we prevent them? God knows we want to prevent them rather than take care of them. I would be delighted to put myself out of the spinal cord injury business tomorrow if we could eliminate spinal cord injuries just as we have almost eliminated poliomyelitis. Many of you out there remember the days of polio when child after child after child came into our orthopedic clinics with devastating disabilities from poliomyelitis. Thank God they don't come in now. Now we see a different type of disability, some of the neglected things such as spinal cord injury.

I'm going to stop talking now and I'm going to ask the various members of our multi-disciplinary group from our Spinal Cord Injury Center to talk with you.

Note

1. *Editors' Note:* In the Lamar Rehabilitation Center of Baptist Memorial Hospital, Memphis, Tennessee, the spinal cord injured individual is treated in the Spinal Cord Injury Unit by a team effort. Members of the team include the physical therapist, nurse, occupational therapist, orthotist, psychologist, social service worker, chaplain, and vocational rehabilitation counselor. The patient is also considered a member of the team. In the following seven papers, the important aspects of the various disciplines are presented by a representative of each.

Marilyn Starrett

Physical Therapy Role in the Treatment of Spinal Cord Injuries

Physical therapy in the treatment of spinal cord injuries plays a role in the four major areas of evaluation, treatment, selection of equipment for home use, and interaction with other team members. Evaluation of muscle strength, sensory deficit, range of motion, and status of activities in daily living is done before actual treatment is begun. Various treatment procedures, especially those leading to successful transferring, are mentioned. Interaction of all team members is emphasized as being most important.

Good afternoon, ladies and gentlemen. This afternoon I would like to discuss with you the role of physical therapy (PT) in the team approch to spinal cord injuries.

Let me begin by saying there are four major areas that I would like to talk about. The first area is the evaluation. It is necessary for us to know exactly what the patient has going for him in order to determine what our individual treatment plan and goals will be. The first part of our evaluation is a muscle test. This is simply judging the strength of the patient's muscles, assigning them a grade, and recording it on a chart. By retesting later on in the course of treatment, changes in strength can be determined accurately and the treatment changed accordingly. The second part of our evaluation is a sensory test. This is done to determine the amount and areas of sensory deficit. Areas of decreased sensation are subject to pressure sores and the skin must be observed carefully. The third section of our evaluation is a range of motion test. This determines if there is any joint tightness or contracture present and to what degree. Lack of proper joint motion may limit the patient's activities and must be improved as much as possible.

If the patient is an old injury, that is, if he has been up in a wheel-chair and moving about, we evaluate the status of his activities of daily living. For example, can he transfer? If so, what type of transfer does he use? How well does he do it? Does he need help?

181

Once all of these tests are done a summary of the findings is written. This summary also includes our treatment plan and goals and is presented with the other team reports to Dr. Tooms. After this discussion, the team members meet with the patient and his family to discuss the report. We feel that the patient is the most important part of the team and must know from the beginning what we expect from him and what he can expect from us.

The second major area I would like to discuss is the actual treatment of the patient. A series of slides will be used to illustrate some of the procedures involved here. Once clearance has been obtained from the physician, one of the first procedures that is begun is the tilt table. Slide one shows a patient utilizing this table. Patients who have been bedridden for a length of time and have loss of muscle tone due to spinal cord injury do not tolerate the upright position. By using this table and gradually bringing the patient to an upright position his tolerance can be increased. Bearing weight on the bones helps decrease loss of calcium and thereby decreases the chance of formation of kidney and bladder stones. Psychologically, the patient benefits from looking at the world from a straight-on position rather than flat on his back.

We also begin strengthening exercises for the muscles that are functioning. This can be accomplished by manual resistance of the therapist, or, as shown in slide two, by the use of weights. Maximum strength of all functioning muscles is a must if the patient is to achieve any degree of independence. Unfortunately, many of these patients have few muscles functioning, so it is mandatory that they attain the best possible use of them. The type of strengthening exercise is determined individually, of course, and a varied combination of techniques may be used.

Besides the maximum strength that we try to attain, there is also a minimum amount of joint motion that we need for certain activities. Slide three illustrates the range of motion exercise that must be done by the therapist to maintain this range. A certain amount of selective stretching in tightened areas is also necessary to gain motion. For example, a certain amount of hip motion is necessary to allow the patient to learn dressing techniques taught by occupational therapy.

Once the patient has attained sufficient strength and spine stability more vigorous activities are begun on the mat. Slide four shows the therapist working on the patient's sitting balance. Learning how to roll over, come to a sitting position, and to move about on the bed are all prerequisite to transfering or to the OT activities of dressing or bathing.

Transfers, or the techniques of getting oneself from one place to another, are a major part of the physical therapy program. There are several types of transfers, and it depends on the patient's strength and balance as to which he can accomplish. Slide five illustrates the swivel bar transfer. This method uses one person to lift the patient's feet and swing him into the chair while the patient hangs on to the overhead bar. This transfer the patient cannot do independently, but it is easier on the assistant than having to pick him up bodily.

The next slide shows a patient getting into a car using a slide board. The board is smooth and polished and very slick. This enables the patient to slide across the board with a minimum of effort. If the patient is strong enough he can do away with assistive equipment and lift himself from the chair with a shoulder depression movement.

Unfortunately, only a small percentage of our patients can benefit from what slide seven is showing: gait training. This patient is using long leg braces in the parallel bars as practice before he progresses to crutches. It has been our experience that only those patients whose injuries are low thoracic or lumbar level and who have functioning muscles around their hips really become functional in their walking. By functional I mean using their braces and crutches a large percentage of the time to do work. Patients with higher injuries do learn to use braces and crutches, but we have found that the large amount of energy expended makes it impractical for everyday getting about.

The third major area in which physical therapy gets involved is the selection of equipment for home use. Of all of the equipment that a patient might need, I suppose the most important is the wheelchair. A wheelchair takes the place of legs that do not work and provides needed mobility. Because the patient often spends many hours in his wheelchair, it is of vital importance that it be the proper one for that person. Wheelchairs come in many sizes, widths, and heights, with many different accessories and attachments, and so it is necessary that the chair be prescribed by the therapist or physician with knowledge of the particular situation.

The next slide shows a hydraulic lift that is used to move the severely disabled from bed to chair or car. It is an important part of our job to assist families in selecting the proper equipment for the home and in making the necessary home adaptations to accomodate the patient.

The last major area that involves physical therapy is the interaction with other team members to make a successful team effort. This is probably the most important area of all because each one of us alone cannot be successful without the help of the others. For example, there are three areas in nursing that can effect the success of a physical therapy program. Proper care and regulation of the bowel and bladder are necessary for a physically healthy patient, and elimination of the embarrassment of accidents is necessary for an emotionally healthy one. Patients must learn proper skin care also, for open pressure sores are a source of infection and a hindrance to a rehabilitation program. The physical therapy department also depends on nursing for coordination of our efforts and for follow-up to see that certain procedures are practiced.

Perhaps occupational therapy (OT) and physical therapy (PT) are more closely related than any of the other team members. Both strengthen muscles, mobilize joints, and teach activities of daily living techniques. Occupational therapy teaches the basic self-care functions of feeding, bathing and dressing, and we depend on them for that. But OT depends on physical therapy, too, for development of adequate balance and strength in the patients so they can accomplish their tasks.

Proper fabrication of hand splints and braces is necessary for the patient to achieve maximum use of his abilities. We rely on the orthotist for advice on special adaptive equipment and special problems of bracing that occur.

We depend on the psychologist to assess the patient's intellectual abilities and personality characteristics. This assists the staff in knowing if the patient can understand, remember, and follow instructions. It also assists them in knowing how to approach and establish rapport with the patient. The psychologist is also invaluable in counseling the patient.

Social service contacts the family, finds out about the home situation, and assists with financial problems and the purchase of equipment. The social service department, along with the chaplain, also counsels with the patient and the family, assisting them in acceptance of the disability and in solving the accompanying problems.

Last, but certainly not least, is the vocational rehabilitation counselor. Our department depends largely on vocational rehabilitation for sponsorship and equipment purchase. We are fortunate enough to have our own counselor who makes rounds with us regularly. She is invaluable as a liason with out of town counselors and as a source of advice as to what the patient will be doing after discharge and that the result of our work will be employment.

Nursing Aspects of the Program

The specialities which nursing training brings to the spinal cord injury patient greatly increase his life expectancy. He is taught how to deal with bodily functions and to assume responsibility for his care. Correct procedures for preventing pressure sores are delineated. This frequently encountered complication is extremely expensive in terms of money, time, and pain. Rehabilitation procedures taught by nursing can free a member of the patient's family for employment even though the patient himself may not be able to resume work.

Where does the nurse fit in the team concept of rehabilitation? The nurse has the responsibility to maintain life, establish good health hygiene, assist the individual to adjust and cope, coordinate the acquired physical and occupational therapy skills on the unit, establish realistic goals, make daily assessments, counsel, prevent complications, communicate and consult with team members, establish safety precautions, bridge the gap from hospital to community, and teach. The specialties that nursing has to offer your client will increase life expectancy as opposed to the prognosis of spinal cord injury years ago. Such catastrophic injury changes all bodily functions. Functions that most of us take for granted must be dealt with on a daily, realistic, and conscientious basis.

I would like to discuss John Doe as an example. He worked diligently in physical and occupational therapy in order to become independent. He was so *gung ho* that he spent the greater part of the day in therapy working with weights. Well motivated, right? On the ward he was too fatigued to give time to bowel or bladder training. He was personable and could usually manipulate some staff member into performing care which was his responsibility. John was fortunate to have an employer who was keeping his former position open until the time he could return to work. Eventually, John returned to work, living in constant fear and anxiety due to humiliating incontinent bowel movements. He was unable to accept social invitations or participate in civic matters which he so enjoyed before injury. Then

187

there were those frequent urinary tract infections which necessitated repeated hospitalization and absences from work. In his zeal to make up lost time, he failed to decompress and soon developed a pressure sore which could not be resolved other than through surgery. Surgical correction meant ten weeks away from work. Needless to say, John subsequently lost his employment and it could have been prevented. This is what it is all about! Skills acquired in the therapy departments are to no avail without learning and assuming responsibility for the body functions while in the rehabilitation center.

Training the bowels is a basic and simple procedure but definitely unique on the cord unit. I read through the nursing records from the acute center and find an enema was given resulting in the inability of the patient to retain the solution. I want to laugh, but it really is not humorous. Of course the patient cannot retain the solution; the rectal sphincter is paralyzed the same as the leg muscles. On the spinal cord unit, enemas are given as a last resort, for repeated enemas will distend the colon and result in loss of bowel tone with ineffectual evacuation. The bowel program is adjusted for each individual but basically requires a mild laxative or prune juice, stool softener suppository, digital stimulation, and primarily a regular schedule. In teaching the patient or family member the bowel procedure, it is frequently heard that brother, sister or Aunt Hattie has worked in the local hospital and given many suppositories; suffice it to say that inserting a suppository is not all there is to it. An established bowel program allows one to feel well, maintain dignity, and, most importantly, protects the skin.

Bladder training is accomplished in a variety of ways. Bladder training is in actuality allowing the bladder to fill and empty on a controlled basis in order to maintain normal tone. Numerous complications arise secondary to an indwelling catheter. The patient is prone to bladder infections, stone formation, epidimytis and penoscrotal fistula, to name a few. All endeavors are made to achieve a catheter-free status. If reflex voiding is not spontaneously established, the urologist is having a great degree of success by performing a transureteral resection and spincterotomy. The long-term prognosis is greatly enhanced by eliminating the complications associated with the indwelling catheter, to say nothing of reducing time and cost involved to the client.

Speaking of cost, I would like to give you the inside track on how to save $7,000. One pressure sore is said to cost this amount. It is therefore sound reasoning to see that your potential client is moved at the earliest possible date to a rehabilitation center where prevention of complications is the rule as opposed to the exception. The clients we are presently receiving indicate an improvement in the quality of nursing care given in the acute center, but the problem has in no way been eliminated. Pressure ulcer is a frequently encountered complication of the spinal cord individual. Simplicity of definition, as indicated by the term, means an ulcer created by pressure. Ulcer formation may begin in a matter of hours and, when allowed to progress, will require a resolution period of several months. An ulcer will begin over any bony prominence which bears weight. With prolonged weight bearing, circulation is eliminated and the shearing force of the bone destroys cells. When cell destruction occurs, tissue death follows. It begins as an innocent appearing red spot. That red spot is calling out, "STOP! KEEP OFF!" It is like the warning stop sign you see every day when driving your automobile. Ignore the red spot and in a brief span of time the warning signal has progressed to necrosis with sloughing. Perhaps it can be resolved by conservative treatment, meaning no surgery. The treatment will consist of scrubbing with a germicidal agent, topical medication, dressings two or more times daily, and—of paramount importance—no pressure. Nine times out of ten, no pressure means the client is confined to the bed and is therefore unable to attend therapy. A pressure ulcer is likened to an iceberg in that only one-third of the involved tissue is visible while the remaining two-thirds is below the surface. By virtue of poor nursing care, the area can progress to the point of bone necrosis. An irreversable situation has developed and will require surgical correction. Before surgery is possible, the area must be debrided of all necrotic tissue either mechanically or by debriding enzymatic agents and, most often, a combination of the two. Due to extensive tissue loss and poor circulation, the prognosis of surgical closure is extremely guarded. Postoperative, the patient requires a period of immobilization of six to ten weeks; that is, providing everything goes well. During this time the client faces the prospect of possible loss of strength, loss of muscle function, possible development of contractures, and valuable loss of physical and occupational therapy time. All are vital in the progressive rehabilitation process. The need for prevention becomes quite evident. Prevention is simple and need not require sophisticated or expensive equipment. Relief of pressure requires a strict turning schedule every two hours when the patient is in bed and frequent decompression when sitting in a wheelchair.

The client must be educated and motivated to assume full responsibility for his own care. The high level quadraplegic may be unable to perform all self-care but is responsible for learning to ask assistance and being able to give detailed directions for his care.

Vocational rehabilitation sponsors a client with the concept of his return to work. This does not always materialize. Rehabilitation does free an able bodied member of the family to work and the client to avoid complications. This is successful sponsorship and rehabilitation.

Occupational Therapy

Occupational therapy functions not only in the role ascribed to it by the general public—that of exploring avocational and prevocational interests—but also with goals of increasing upper extremity strength and function, helping the patient to achieve independence in daily living, and making evaluations for orthotic and adaptive equipment.

Occupational therapy's role as a member in the spinal cord injury team includes increasing upper extremity strength and function, helping the patient to achieve independence in activities of daily living, making recommendations for splints and splint training, and exploring avocational and prevocational interests.

When the patient is admitted to the center, he is given a complete evaluation. This includes:

1. Upper extremity strength—manual muscle test to note functioning muscles and their strength.
2. U.E. Range of Motion—notes any limitation in degrees of movement each joint goes through.
3. U.E. Sensation—tests for sharp-dull (pain), temperature, object identification, and proprioception (joint motion).
4. Activities of Daily Living—self care, homemaking and other living skills (dressing, feeding, functional communication, transportation, etc.)
5. Splinting—evaluate any U.E. orthotic equipment he presently has and evaluate the need for such equipment.
6. Adaptive Equipment—evaluate for adaptive equipment which may be needed in the future for independence in self-care skills or homemaking; examples are special eating utensils or button hooks.
7. Prevocational and avocational interests.

The team then has a staff conference to discuss findings and explore the needs of the patient. We then meet with the patient and

191

his family. The patient is one of the most important members of the team, and this gives him the opportunity to discuss our findings and goals for him and goals he has set for himself.

The treatment is based on the initial evaluation. Range of motion may have to be increased through passive stretching and/or positional splinting. Upper extremity muscles may need strengthening in order to have the active range of motion and endurance necessary for independence in self-care skills. This strength may be gained through progressive resistive exercises (weights, etc.), activities selected for their resistive exercise (crafts, self-care skills), or games (punching bags, volleyball, ping-pong). Most strengthening OT is done sitting in the wheelchair rather than on the mat as in PT. The patient needs to learn to maintain balance and still make functional use of his arms.

The patient must be taught precautions concerning loss of sensation to body parts. He must become aware of the dangers of injuring extremities with impaired sensation. This includes inspection for red spots caused by unrelieved pressure as in sitting.

Each patient is encouraged to reach his highest potential in self-care independence. This may require hours of long hard work, special adaptive equipment, and orthotic devices. If need be, the patient is seen in feeding class and/or dressing class besides his daily clinic treatment.

Many times splints are recommended. Positioning splints are necessary to protect weak muscles or stretch out contractures. Dynamic splints are usually recommended for those who have no prehension or whose hand strength is too weak for functional use. The decision on choice of splinting is made by evaluating the patient's strength, hand placement, motivation, intelligence, and gadget tolerance. Examples of this include the need for wrist extensors strong enough to operate the wrist driven flexor hinge splint. The patient who does not have wrist extension but has good hand placement may be fitted with a ratchet splint. He should be able to put it on and take it off independently and position objects to be used in it. If the patient can not handle a ratchet splint we may consider an externally powered splint such as a harness or an electric powered one. When fitting this expensive, technical equipment one must very closely evaluate the patient's ability to understand the proper care and use of the equipment and the motivation to use it, in addition to the items mentioned previously. With the above mentioned splints, most patients can feed themselves, brush their teeth, shave, put on makeup, type, play some games (checkers, cards, etc.), and do some writing. In OT we check to see that splints are fitting correctly and that the patient is trained to use them functionally.

Homemaking skills are explored with all patients who have the muscle function necessary to perform the activities. Women will need to know how to function in their kitchens at home. Male patients may need to know some homemaking skills when they go to school, live in an apartment, or are possibly left at home with children while the wife assumes the role of the major income person.

Basic prevocational skills are often explored. We don't, however, do prevocational evaluations but often refer patients to an evaluation center in the area.

In closing, occupational therapy is just one member of the team. We could not function adequately without the other members' contributions.

The Use of Extended Evaluation
in Serving the Severely Disabled

Benefits of extended evaluation services are described. Guidelines for their use are set forth, and listings of services which can and cannot be provided are given.

As you know, the 1965 amendments to the Vocational Rehabilitation Act provide to us the use of extended evaluation services, status 06, when we are unable to determine the vocational potential of individuals whose disabilities fall into certain categories. Certainly with the coming of the 1973 amendments this status should prove to be of additional value as more and more severely disabled individuals are being identified and referred to us.

To refresh our memories, let's review what services can and cannot be provided to clients placed in this status. We can provide counseling and guidance, physical restoration, maintenance and transportation, training and training materials, reader services for the blind, interpreter services for the deaf, comprehensive evaluation at a rehabilitation facility, and other services which are necessary to determine vocational potential. Since all these services are diagnostic in scope, it is not necessary to consider economic need, if your state is one which considers this.

Services which cannot be provided are placement and/or placement tools, occupational licenses, and management services and supervision for vending stand or other small business enterprises.

Counselors may be reluctant to use extended evaluation services since it may be necessary to write two plans for some individuals—I hope for many, many individuals! And, also, at this time we receive little or no credit for our efforts when using this status. Perhaps this will change in the numbers game." We hope!

But certainly there are also advantages in using this status when working with severely disabled individuals. As a counselor assigned to the Lamar Unit of Baptist Memorial Hospital in Memphis, I am involved primarily with Spinal Cord Injured patients, although severe arthritic patients, stroke and hemodialysis patients are also referred to us. We are considered to be a member of a rehabilitation team concerned with the total rehabilitation of these severely disabled patients. Our plans are written for extended evaluation. With the assistance of other team members, we can make a determination of a patient's vocational potential. Certainly, being a member of such a team is a unique and valuable experience and an advantage when working with severely disabled!

Again, I would like to urge your consideration of extended evaluation services when working with severely disabled individuals.

The Role of the Orthotist

The orthotist in recent years has seen improvements in lower extremity bracing in three areas: cosmesis, increased function, and reduced bulk. Great progress has been made in providing or enhancing upper extremity function. Prehension type orthotic devices include the wrist driven flexor hinge splint, ratchet driven tenodesis splint, and the externally powered tenodesis splint, of which there are two basic types. Individual decisions as to the most appropriate type must be made.

The role of the orthotist, in the team concept, is to measure, design, fabricate, and fit orthotic systems for the severely disabled spinal cord injured patient. In the early stages of the injury, this bracing is confined to supporting the damaged portion of the spine by means of cervical or spinal bracing. Bracing of the extremities is begun as the patient moves into the rehabilitation phase of his treatment.

The paraplegic patient who has a relatively low lesion and some voluntary control of his hip musculature can ambulate with the assistance of bilateral long leg braces. It is difficult, if not impossible, for adults with lesions of a slightly higher level to ambulate with full control braces (a full control brace being bilaterial long leg braces with pelvic band and spinal brace attachment). However, children with high lesions are quite often able to ambulate with the assistance of full control braces.

In recent years, lower extremity bracing has been improved considerably in three areas: cosmesis, increased function, and reduced bulk of the orthotic device. So far as cosmesis is concerned, the addition of plastics into the orthotic field has been a tremendous help toward improved cosmetic appearance. Some of the new orthotic devices, especially below knee devices, can be fabricated entirely of plastic, resulting in not only a cosmetically superior item, but a much lighter weight orthotic device. In our more conventional metal bracing we are covering the metal uprights with a vinyl material that is available in a variety of fleshtone colors. This renders the device not only cosmetically more acceptable, but also protects the patient's clothing from the metal parts and is impervious to urine.

Through investigation of the principles that we have used in our prosthetic fabrication for a number of years, we have been able to apply these principles to leg bracing in order to produce a more functional brace with less bulk. In many instances we are able to fit a patient with a short leg brace, whereas he would have previously required a long leg brace to achieve the same degree of control. Incorporating these prosthetic principles not only allows us to use a modified short leg brace, but also to do away with the requirement for knee locks in some cases. Ambulation without knee locks is easier, as is going from a sitting to a standing position, or vice versa.

The patient who has been rendered quadriplegic presents the orthotist with an entirely different problem. The problem is primarily related to providing, or enhancing, upper extremity function. The orthotist, through conventional style hand splinting, and in consultation with the therapist, designs and fits positioning type hand splints that are used in the initial stages to prevent unwanted flexion contractures and to maintain the positive results gained by the patient through therapy programs.

Later in the rehabilitation stage, the quadriplegic has a need for prehension type orthotic devices. These devices have to be customized by the orthotist to take advantage of whatever remaining function the patient might have. For example, the patient often will have wrist motion, but no finger motion. In this case, the orthotist could fabricate a wrist driven flexor hinge splint, which would provide the patient with the necessary prehension force by harnessing the motion remaining at the wrist joint. There are numerous variations of this splint that the orthotist might use, depending upon the functional deficit. If there is no wrist motion available, a more sophisticated system can be used. For example, a ratchet driven tenodesis splint can be closed pasively by the patient on any object that he wishes to hold. The ratchet mechanism will prevent the object from falling out of the splint. By touching a release button the object can then be released. In addition to the passively powered ratchet splint, it is sometimes possible to body power the same type of splint with a control cable similar to that used in an upper extremity prosthesis.

If the patient has no body power source to harness, it is possible to use an externally powered tenodesis splint. There are two basic types of these splints. One is electrically powered by a rechargeable nickel-cadium battery. By the mere touch of a micro-switch with any portion of the body, such as head, opposite hand, shoulder elevation or even in some cases a tongue switch, finger prehension is provided. The other externally powered system available is a CO_2 system which incorporates the use of an artificial muscle whereby the patient can open or close a valve similar to the way he operates the micro-switch on the electric splint. By opening and closing the valve, he can introduce gas into the artificial muscle causing it to shorten and close the fingers, or expel gas from the artificial muscle causing it to elongate and open the fingers.

The advantage of the CO_2 system is that it provides some proportional control. It is possible for the patient to crack the valve open slightly and have a slow closure of the fingers or open the valve fully and have a fairly rapid closure of the fingers. The electrical system is a one speed system; the switch is either on or off. There are, however, in the design stages some proportionally controlled electrical systems that will accomplish the same type of operation that we alluded to in the CO_2 system. The obvious advantage of the electrical system over the CO_2 is the ease of recharging the nickel-cadium battery by plugging it into the wall overnight. The availability of a home supply to recharge CO_2 cylinders is cumbersome, expensive, and difficult, if not impossible, for the patient to manage.

In summary, the orthotist, in close consultation with the physical and occupational therapist, works closely to evaluate the patient's functional deficit and recommends to the prescribing physician what he feels would be the most appropriate orthotic systems for each individual patient.

Ronald J. Karney

Psychosocial Aspects of the Spinal Cord Injured: The Psychologist's Approach

The psychologist reviews the stages of adjustment through which the patient passes and the important roles the rehabilitation center and psychologist play in this psychosocial adjustment. Information and counseling in the areas of sexual life, abilities, and necessary adjustments of the spinal cord injured patient are felt to be most important in the rehabilitation of the individual. Contributions of the psychologist to the team approach are in three main areas: evaluation, counseling, and staff consultation.

This talk and the following two presentations deal with the psychosocial aspects of the rehabilitation of the spinal cord injured (SCI) individual. This area of the SCI's adjustments is complex, and no one discipline holds the key or magic formula to help every patient. At Lamar Unit we realize this and have three primary disciplines that deal with the psychosocial adjustment, as well as a team approach that integrates this aspect within the daily treatment of our clients.

This talk primarily deals with the psychologist's approach at Lamar Unit and will cover the following points: stages of adjustment, sexual adjustment, how the rehabilitation center is important for psychosocial adjustment, and the role of the psychologist.

STAGES OF ADJUSTMENT

At Lamar Unit we follow the theoretical model of adjustment conceptualized by Fink for traumatic, catastrophic disabilities such as a spinal cord injury. This model allows us to determine where an individual is when he comes to the center, what must be done to help him move forward, what we can expect, and where he will be located upon discharge. According to this model, every patient must pass through each stage, although they will vary in the length of time each one will stay in each stage. Let us briefly review each of the four stages of adjustment:

201

1. *Shock.* In this stage the individual realizes danger or threat and has feelings of fear and helplessness. He may appear totally overcome by his disability and may be disoriented. The individual experiences only partial awareness of what has happened and what is being done. We rarely receive individuals within this stage because of the nature of our rehabilitation center and the time it takes to get here. The majority of patients experience this stage while they are in other hospitals recovering from the immediate physical shock to their bodies.

2. *Defensive Retreat or Denial.* Here the individual becomes aware of what has happened and employs defense mechanisms to protect himself from the reality of his situation. The most common defense mechanisms are rationalization and denial. Most of our clients come to our center in this stage of their adjustment. This stage is probably the most difficult to deal with because the individual can easily bolster his defenses and avoid dealing with the reality of his situation by selective inattention.

   At the rehabilitation center we attempt to undermine these defenses by using a realistic approach with the individual which may be considered "cruel" by members of his family should they try to employ it. In our approach we deal with the reality of the present and do not reinforce statements made by the individual which appear unrealistic. Also, the environment of the center is important in preventing the buildup of denial. More will be said about the environment later.

   Although I have no empirical evidence for this statement, I have noted that some of the most difficult individuals with whom we work have been typically discharged from the hospital, sent home for many months to several years, and then brought to the center. During this time their degree of denial becomes so strong that it is very difficult to help them move into the next stage of adjustment.

3. *Acknowledgment and Depression.* The individual becomes consciously aware of the permanence of his disability and his loss of a previous way of life. This stage is typically characterized by depression, which is a healthy sign in that it shows that the individual has entered into this phase of adjustment. During this stage attention shifts from undermining the individual's defenses to

providing supportive therapy in order to help him work through his depression.

4. *Adaptation.* The individual begins adjusting to his disability by reordering his priorities. Reality contact is good, and he becomes motivated toward total rehabilitation.

The Rehabilitation Center is important is helping the individual work through these stages primarily by providing a safe, conducive environment. This environment consists of:

1. Other patients who have a similar type of disability and who are at different stages in their adjustment. The more advanced patients give support, encouragement, and a realistic orientation to the newly arrived individuals. At times the advanced patients will blast unrealistic statements a patient may make and help him acknowledge that they are unrealistic.
2. The clients at the center live in an environment that deals with the realities of the moment. Patients are given feedback by their therapists about any improvement or lack of improvement. They can examine the progress they have made as well as the plateaus they have reached. The patients are required to perform activities that they are capable of and are not permitted to slack off and wait for that day of their hopeful, total, functional return. By dealing with such realities the individual is not given the opportunity to avoid them and strengthen his denial.
3. Professional staff are available for individual psychotherapy, family therapy, and group therapy in order to deal with rationalizations and other defense mechanisms that may impede the individuals progress toward adjustment.

Such an environment cannot be adequately established if the individual lives at home with his family and friends who may feel "sorry" for him and thus avoid dealing with the realities of the moment. In addition, the degree of emotional involvement they have with the SCI individual may inhibit their ability to deal with the reality of the situation.

SEXUAL ADJUSTMENT

Take a moment and answer this question: "Does a SCI individual have a sexual life?" In all probability the majority of people have answered either "No," or "I've never thought of that." This area of functioning has been sorely neglected for many years, and most of the information that the average person has about this area is based upon stereotyped attitudes toward the physically disabled as being asexual creatures. Yet this is one area of functioning that many SCI individuals wish to find answers about. They want to know if their sexual lives will be affected as a result of their injury.

The answer to the question I asked is "Yes!" A sexual life for the SCI does exist and is guided by the principle of doing whatever is physiologically and psychologically feasible. In physiological terms this may be anything from touching to intercourse, depending upon the level of injury. In psychological terms it may be whatever is aesthetically pleasing to both partners and not against the morals and values of the individual.

Let us briefly review the physiological abilities of both the male and female SCI. (Slide). The male's sexual organs depend upon neurological intervention. As a result there may be some impairment of the male's ability to obtain an erection, maintain it through intercourse, and produce progeny. As you can see there are two types of erections possible: (1) reflexogenic with upper motor neuron (UMN) lesions, which is a spontaneous or physically stimulated erection, and (2) psychogenic with lower motor neuron (LMN) lesions, which is psychologically produced. These statistics tell us that the majority of male SCI individuals can engage in sexual intercourse. However, we must deal with each individual in a nonstatistical manner. Figures are not available about individuals engaging in other forms of sexual activities, but they are probably much higher because of the ease in engaging in them. The sexual organs of the SCI female are not dependent upon neurological intervention, except for sensation, and as a result they are capable of all forms of sexual expression as well as being able to become pregnant.

At Lamar Unit we are aware of this areas of adjustment and provide counseling as well as an atmosphere in which discussion about sex is not frowned upon but encouraged. Our philosophy about sex centers around the following points:

1. It is a necessary part of human functioning, being the expression of a human emotion in a multitude of ways, provided they are compatible with the patient's morals and values.

2. Discussion is encouraged, and an environment is provided that is open and conducive to this goal.
3. We are sensitive to an individual's feelings about sex and do not force him or her into discussing sexual adjustment. Instead, we inform each about the opportunity to engage in counseling both alone and with a partner.
4. We are honest and realistic in the information we provide and take care to help the individual discover what is feasible and the necessary precautions which are important.

This area of adjustment is important to the individual's self concept of being male or female, and we attempt to provide this service to every one of our clients. Such information is not readily available for the SCI individual who remains at home in at attempt to deal with his rehabilitation alone. This is one service which our center can offer to round out the entire, total rehabilitation of the SCI individual.

ROLL OF THE PSYCHOLOGIST

At Lamar Unit the psychologist is just one member of a well-functioning team. Although there is some overlap with some of the other disciplines, the major contributions can be broken down into three areas:

1. *Evaluative.* Psychological evaluations are given to every individual upon admission to our unit. In this evaluation we are looking for the person's intellectual level, stage of adjustment, and conflicts that may impede the patient's total rehabilitation should they go unresolved. This evaluation helps the other staff members in formulating a group approach to working with an individual which is compatible with his abilities and personality.
2. *Counseling.* Individual, family, and group therapy are provided in order to help the individual in his adjustment. Sexual adjustment is an important aspect which is covered through individual and marital counseling.
3. *Consulting.* In this role the psychologist helps the staff in dealing with patients who may be difficult to work with and also provides inservice training on the psychological dynamics of the SCI.

Bob Klutts

The Chaplain's Ministry to the
Spinal Cord Injury Patient

The chaplain plays an active role in the team approach to treatment of the spinal cord injured patient because many adjustment problems arise due to inadequate religious backgrounds. Typical religious problems are listed with the basic types of ministries offered for each. The chaplain relates in different ways to the various stages of adjustment (described by the psychologist) as the patient passes through each. Focus is on redirecting the patient's life and reinforcing a positive image of self-worth.

In dealing with the spinal cord injured patient the chaplain adds a pastoral perspective to the treatment of the patient, and he also adds pastoral authority in relating to the patient. The latter is certainly as important as the first. Both derive their importance from the fact that many of the problems that the patient has in his development and adjustment come from an inadequate religious background. This means he needs someone who can relate to his religious needs. As a minister I can speak to him with a religious authority that the other team members do not have. Many of the things he uses to deny what the future hold for him and will demand from him come from the fact that his religious leader often has told him, "Anything is possible if you have faith." As a minister the chaplain tries to communicate that many things are just the way they are, they will stay the way they are, and one has to make the best of things under the limitations that exist. This is a realistic approach that deals with the religious needs of the patient as well as reinforces the efforts of the rest of the team members.

TYPICAL RELIGIOUS PROBLEMS

1. *Crisis Experience.* It is important to keep in mind that the patient has had a very severe crisis experience. Any crisis experience is a crisis in the person's religious life. This means that his religious concerns are heightened and that his whole world in a sense has

207

been transformed. Everything is upside down; things are not the way they were. Even though he has had a very strong religious background it probably isn't able to meet his needs at first. If he had a weak religious background, many times he becomes far more religious than he ever was before, but many times that new-found religion is unhealthy and will hurt his rehabilitation.

2. *Guilt.* One of the common religious concerns is the patient's feeling of guilt. He often feels that God is paying him back for some bad thing he has done. When he sees the injury as punishment he needs to have a feeling of forgiveness and acceptance. He needs to know not only that I accept him, but that God accepts him so he can get over the idea that God is punishing him for something he has done.

3. *Miracle.* Linked with this idea of guilt is the feeling that a miracle is going to happen to him. Many of the patients see themselves as being the exception: a miracle is going to happen to them. Maybe to no one else, but they are the ones who are going to walk out of the building in as good a shape as they were before their injuries. The chaplain tries to help them deal with this idea and show them that they have to face life as it is; they have to adjust to life as it is. Along with this they also need to have a feeling of hope and a sense of God's involvement in their life. Things are not all over for them even though things physically most likely will not improve a tremendous amount, and certainly not as much as they wish. They need to adjust their ideas of how God is involved in their lives.

4. *Readjustment of Values.* There is a major readjustment of values in their lives. The chaplain tries to give some guidance as they try to re-establish their priorities—what really are the most important things in their lives. They have to do this whether they like it or not if life is going to be positive and worth living. There seem to be a million things they can no longer do, so they need to find some system of values that will give them a meaning and purpose in life.

5. *Need to Affirm Themselves and Life.* They also have the need to affirm themselves and their lives. The patient needs to see himself as a person who has value. Many times a patient will look at himself, think of what he once could do and think of what he can no longer do, and say his life is useless, hopeless, and has no value.

He says, "I am a burden and that is all I am." He needs to find that his life has value and has purpose and meaning. This means that the chaplain focuses on the business of finding self-fulfillment and self-worth.

BASIC TYPES OF MINISTRY

Chaplains try to deal with some of the deepest concerns and needs that the patient has. It is important to focus on a goal that is realistic, but this is just what is often very hard for him to accept.

1. *Focus on Interdependency.* The patient needs to see what is realistic independence as well as realistic dependence in life. Each one of us is both dependent as well as independent to some extent. The patient needs to see that there are some things that are adequate and appropriate along both of these lines for him. He needs to be independent as much as he can, but he also needs to accept the dependence which will be a part of his life from now on. So he needs to come to some consciousness of his unique value and capabilities.

2. *Comfort.* The chaplain tries to bring comfort by empathizing with the patient. He needs assurance, support, and acceptance. The chaplain does not try to tell him, "Have faith and everything will be all right," for things will not be all right. But he does need to accept himself and feel accepted by others, and this can enable him to see that things are not quite the total disaster they appear to be.

3. *Catalytic Agent.* The chaplain serves as a catalytic agent as he tries to help the patient work through the stages of development that our psychologist mentioned in his presentation. I try to accelerate the acceptance that the patient feels for himself and his situation. I try to help him become aware of his capabilities as well as his responsibilities, and both of these are very important for him as they are for everyone. The patient can very easily feel that he can do nothing, and so nothing should be expected of him. But your life and mine derive a lot of their meaning not only from what we are able to do, but also from what we accept as our responsibility and our duty to accomplish.

4. *Challenge.* I try to challenge the patient as he tries to find a new system of values and help him actualize that system of ideas. It is

one thing for him to say, "Yes, life can be meaningful." It is another for him to readjust to what is possible or to what is satisfying. However, unless he accepts those values and commits himself to them and sticks by them, he will have one more failure to live with; so I try to challenge him to commit himself to these positive new values that he has accepted. Then of course he needs his daily progress reinforced.

STAGES OF DEVELOPMENT

1. *Shock.* At the time the patient is experiencing shock the chaplain can be with the patient, be concerned and accepting, provide emotional support, and that's about it.
2. *Denial.* As the patient enters the stage of denial, the chaplain focuses on realism. He reinforces the facts. This does not mean that he is being pushy. It does not mean that he is forcing it down his throat, because the patient may need to deny things to some extent so he can handle them. Still, the chaplain works to bring about a realistic frame of mind.
3. *Acknowledgement.* During the stage of denial, the chaplain helps him work through some of the grief that there is an any time of mourning over a loss. There is a lot of grief involved. When a person loses a part of his body he has in a very realistic sense lost something very important to him, perhaps even as important as many people are to him. His grief can be as severe as the grief over a lost loved one. He must deal with it if he is to work through it. Depression sets in as he begins to fully acknowledge the reality of his situation, and this is a time when he neds a lot of support.
3. *Adjustment.* When the patient reaches the point of adjustment the chaplain reinforces the positive image of self-worth that he is trying to find for himself. I focus on the redirection of his life. I try to help him find some meaning in life regardless of what his situation is going to be. In terms of a dismissal goal, basically what I am trying to do is help the patient have faith in himself and find meaning in life along with having the confidence that God is creatively involved in his life.

The Social Worker's Involvement in the Rehabilitation of the Spinal Cord Injured Individual

The crisis of a spinal cord injury requires many services other than medical. The role of the social worker is one of "social bracing." There are many times during the stay of the patient in the Spinal Cord Injury Center when the social worker is needed to deal with concerns, feelings, worries, and fears of the patient and his family. During discharge planning he must be concerned with assisting the patient in obtaining as high a level of functioning as possible in each area of his life which was significant to him before the injury. These areas may include education/work, marriage/heterosexual relationships, parenthood, religious activities, and leisure time/recreational activities. Most important is the restoration of a feeling of self-worth in the individual and of others' beliefs in his worth. The social worker must think of the client not as a "case," a medical problem, a statistic, or a liability, but as a "whole person."

Ways in which the rehabilitation counselor can continue the work of the social worker and maintain contact with him are listed.

I want to talk to you about the social worker's role as an integral member of the rehabilitation team, just *WHO* he is, *WHAT* he does, *WHEN* and *HOW* he does it and *WHY*. Key words come to mind. I think of "handicapped—disabled" or potentially or temporarily. Someone has provided the following definition: "any disadvantage that renders success more difficult."[1] Then "brace"—to furnish support; to support by providing firmness; to place in a position for resisting pressure.[2] Feelings and attitudes about these two key words color and greatly influence the rehabilitation process of the spinal cord injured individual. The crisis of a spinal cord injury requires all sorts of responses that are other than medical. Let's call the social worker's role "social bracing."

WHO

He is one concerned with responding to the "whole person" to have a healthy person at home as independent as possible because:

211

a successfully rehabilitated person is one who is able to live in a non-medical setting at a level of occupational and social performance comparable with other adults in the community.[3]

In the discharge of his responsibilities, the social worker must make several assumptions. Of the following four the first two relate to the spinal cord injured individual, while the latter relate to the social worker:

1. Changes in self-concept and self-image take place. The spinal cord injured individual will develop different feelings about himself and how he gets along with himself and others.
2. Role changes become evident. Regardless of what roles he took part in, they will be altered. Some degree of new life style will develop because of his physical problems.
3. Each spinal cord injured individual will have to be seen and valued as an individual of worth. Perhaps this can best be seen by the social worker's willingness to foster realistic independence in the spinal cord injured individual.
4. People are capable of change, but they may not change. Spinal cord injured individuals can be difficult individuals to deal with. There may be times when the social worker gets discouraged, perhaps to the point of giving up, or of feeling that the spinal cord injured individual's frustration is being directed toward him and finding it not worth it.

WHAT

When a person suffers a spinal cord injury that creates a temporary or permanent disfunction, he is concerned about what he will or will not be able to do. In order to know *what* to do to aid in his rehabilitation, a social history is obtained to learn about the areas of his life that are/were significant to him prior to his injury. What provided satisfaction, commitment, and dedication are the areas that need "bracing."

Perlman has defined three areas of life that demand our emotional investment.[4] I have added the last two. It is my belief that each of us wears these five "hats" (social roles): (1) education/work, (2)marriage/heterosexual relationships, (3) parenthood, (4) religious activities, and (5) leisure time/recreational activities. When the social worker can learn from the spinal cord injured individual and others involved in his life in these areas, then directions can be focused on assisting him in obtaining as high a level of functioning in each of these roles as possible.

WHEN

When does the spinal cord injured individual need "bracing"? The event of a spinal cord injury is a suprise—a very unwelcome one. The injured and his family are anxious, bewildered, and often immobilized. An effort is made to see both the injured and his family as soon as admission takes place. A bridge/linkage between where they are now and the rehabilitation center is vital in helping them "settle in"; learn about the rehabilitation center and its plans, and how it is different from a hospital. In short, the person and his family should be put at ease so that the rehabilitation process can be as effective as possible.

Another important "when" centers around "discharge planning." Please note that I say discharge planning, not "discharge." This too is a process that enables the social worker and the spinal cord injured individual's family to take an ongoing look at the assets and liabilities/positives and negatives for reassuming his satisfying social roles (the five "hats" mentioned earlier). The "how" of this will be discussed next.

There are many times between the events of admission and discharge when a person and his family need a social worker. Some examples are:

1. dealing with the feelings about having to use a wheelchair, splints or braces, or other adaptive equipment
2. concerns about slow progress or no progress
3. acceptance of physical limitations
4. overdoing or undoing (spinal cord injured individual and/or family)
5. worries/fears
6. discharge planning conferences

The social worker will discuss with the family any adjustments they may need to make to maintain good patient care and maximum independence. This may mean helping them see that caring for their family member may mean "not doing" for him. It means helping them anticipate and deal with problem areas (real or potential) about their family member as well as their own behavior.

HOW

A vital "how" is the utilization of any and all community resources that may be brought to bear on the social roles that the spinal cord injured individual finds significant and on one where he has some degree of functioning. This fosters our concern for the individual and promotes the principle of continuity of care which is essential in the rehabilitation of the spinal cord injured individual.

Maintaining effective communication about treatment with the spinal cord injured individual's sponsor is a necessary factor in the rehabilitation process.

The social worker can approach a tangible task and make a valuable contribution by walking through the door to the intangible. For example, when discussing the purchasing of needed equipment for the spinal cord injured individual, why not deal with the worries and fears he has about the loss of body integrity?

Other "hows" relate to intervention as a team member in the movement through the stages of adjustment as discussed in the papers by the psychologist and chaplain. Treatment goals and aftercare plans can be reinforced. Efforts can be made to negate unrealistic expectations of the spinal cord injured individual and his family.

A spinal cord injured individual truly will have some "disability" and he must be helped to see his "ability."

WHY

Why not? The spinal cord injured individual is not a "case," a medical problem or diagnosis, nor a statistic, nor a liability. *He is one of us with a broken neck or back.* He has all the worries, fears, and concerns about life as do we, and he also has all the goals, ambitions, and aspirations that we do. We want to be useful, wanted, loved, and important—so does the spinal cord injured individual. When the social worker does not respond to the "whole person," rehabilitation can be a disservice.

Why is the social worker such an important factor? Because *he cares*—he cares about what happens to other people. I am convinced by my eleven years in social work that people who *care* can help. It's more than a job; it's a life-long commitment to people. I know that you must care or you wouldn't have assumed the responsibility of your present position.

Because I have nearly four years of experience at a rehabilitation center with vocational rehabilitation counselors of several states, I want to share with you some ideas of how you can "care" for the spinal cord injured individual you are sponsoring.

1. Know the name, address, and phone number of the social worker who is having contact with the spinal cord injured individual you are sponsoring.
2. Maintain the kind of contact with the social worker that you find will aid you in fulfilling your responsibilities. This would include progress notes, phone calls, and letters. Come to see him when you are in town. Make rounds, and attend the planning conferences.
3. Ask questions such as, "What is your understanding of his plans when he is discharged?" and "What sorts of problems does the rehabilitation team anticipate?" Inquire about why the spinal cord injured individual or his family may be anxious about a given aspect.
4. Know the center's treatment plans and goals for the spinal cord injured individuals that you sponsor. Only then can you coordinate your vocational and other plans. The spinal cord injured individual benefits best when his information is known from the very beginning. This process is a good example of responding to the "whole person" and of supporting continuity of care.
5. Keep as up to date as possible about the types of equipment your spinal cord injury clientele will need (wheelchairs—standard or prescription, braces/splints, lifts, and other adaptive equipment) to maximize spinal cord injury independence.
6. Make early referral for physical rehabilitation. Avoid wasting both time and money by purchasing the care that can best help your spinal cord injured clients. Delay can make for physical complications that may be permanent. Delay can keep the spinal

cord injured individual and his family from fostering realistic attitudes and expectations about his physical prowess. Delay can also keep them from overdoing or getting worn out doing for the spinal cord injured individual what he can be taught to do for himself.

7. LeLt the social worker and center hear about your continuing relationship with the spinal cord injured individual after he returns home or goes to another facility in the community.

Notes

1. Henry Bosley Woolf, Editor in Chief, *Webster's New Collegiate Dictionary* (Springfield: G. and C. Merriam Company, 1973), p. 519.

2. *Ibid.,* p. 132.

3. H. E. Freeman and O. G. Simmons, "The Mental Patient Comes Home" (New York: Wiley, 1963) in Silvano Arieti, ed., *American Handbook of Psychiatry,* Vol. III (New York: Basic Books, 1966), p. 645.

4. Helen Harris Perlman, *Social Role and Personality* (Chicago: The University of Chicago Press, 1968), p. 48.

William A. Tomlin

Serving the Severely Disabled

The rehabilitation process is an orderly sequence of services related to the total needs of the handicapped individual and built around the problems of that individual. During this process, the counselor must assume many roles. The addition of the severely disabled to already heavy caseloads increases the types of services needed and their duration.

A "severe handicap" is a disability which requires multiple services over an extended period of time, as a result of any cause. The process of serving these or any other clients is one of three stages—referral, provision of services, and closure. The severely disabled person will have many problems in addition to those of physical restoration, evaluation, training, and job placement. The rehabilitation counselor will find that personal and social situations often require continued counseling after the patient returns home.

Vice President Cliff, President Jenkins, and fellow council members: Cliff, I know you have retired with a great deal of anticipation and have willingly passed over the gavel to Bill Jenkins. I imagine that although your tour as president had its highs, you did experience some lows, and we're now ready to share a great deal of this with you just as a member. Let me say that the Southeast Region once again is number one in NRCA. A great deal of this credit is due to Wayne Mulkey who chaired the regional membership post this year. This year the Southeast Region has experienced, as every state in the region experienced, a significant membership change—an increase. I wish to commend you for your activity.

Many of you have been here all week and you will say, "Well, Bill, you're going to talk about the severely disabled. You know I've heard that all this week." I know you've heard it, but I hope to get it to you in a different manner so that you won't be like a friend of mine in the North Georgia mountains whom I know years ago when we were playing in a championship football game. I was raised in the mountains of North Georgia on the Tennessee-North Carolina line, and our school was classified as a Class C school. This meant that we had fewer than 250 students attending that high school. In the last

217

two or three minutes of the championship game we were behind 13-7. We had the ball, and we were moving towards the goal. Well, as we got nearer the goal, the time started picking up a little faster, and our coach kept saying, "Give the ball to LeRoy." We would run one of our halfbacks into the line, and then they would come out and carry him off the field. The coach was standing on the sideline, and he'd say, "Give the ball to LeRoy." Sure enough ,the quarterback would run another play in the line, and they would come out and carry off another teammate. Well, finally, the coach just walked out and said as loud as he could, "I said, give the damn ball to LeRoy." The quarterback said, "Well, coach, LeRoy says he doesn't want the ball." I think after today some of you may say, "I don't want to hear any more about the severely disabled." However, knowing the dedicated counselors that you are, I hope that what I can give you will help whether you have to continue carrying the ball or not. This is what the counselor does; he carries the ball for the agency. Whatever happens can establish that agency's name as either good or bad. Whatever happens to a client is in your hands because you're carrying the ball for him. This is why I feel that you're still interested in hearing something about the severely disabled.

The rehabilitation process consists of a plan, an orderly sequence of services that are related to the total needs of the handicapped individual. It is a process built around the problems of the handicapped individual. The rehabilitation process attempts to help solve these problems and bring about the vocational rehabilitation of the handicapped or severely impaired person. In this process, the counselor sees himself and his colleagues fulfilling many roles. You sometimes act as a parent. You sometimes act, in a similar manner, as a doctor, a psychologist, a teacher, a policeman, a public relations expert, a personnel manager, or a placement specialist. In reality, you must be a "jack of all trades" in order to ensure that the client receives the best possible services available to him. Our caseloads are heavy, and sometimes you say to your state agency or supervisor, "How can I do any more? I have about 225 persons sitting over here in referred status. I have about 160-175 active cases, and I'm just running to stay alive. Now, you come along ,and you are going to throw another group on us. How do you expect us to do this?"

Sometimes, counselors remind me of the seventy-two-year-old mountain man who was ready to marry for the second time. His children were convinced that he had decided to marry a twenty-six-year-old girl. They didn't know how to counsel their father, because once he had formed an opinion that was it. There was no argument. He had made the decision, and he was going through with it. So they went to see the family physician, and he told them, "Your father is coming in for an examination, and I am going to send him by the Health Department and let him talk with the Family Planning Group." The father went in for the interview and the health nurse who spoke with him said, "Well, sir, you realize what you're getting into." He said "Yes, ma'am, I sure do." She continued, "You are aware of your age," he said, "Yes, ma'am, I sure am." She said, "And you're aware of your wife's age," and he replied, "Yes, ma'am, I sure am." The health nurse said, "Well, really, you might need some help." And the old man said, "Well, you know you're right." The health nurse said to herself, "Well, in just one session of counseling, I have communicated with him." The old man went back home and didn't see the nurse for about six or seven months. She met him one day and asked, "How are you doing?" He said, "Just fine." She said, "And you're married?" He replied, "Oh, yes, my wife is pregnant," She said "Well, what about the help you brought in?" The old man replied, "Oh, she's pregnant too." Well, this is the way we feel sometimes with our caseloads. Often, we feel doubly pregnant, if that is possible, because there is so much emphasis on service to every client you're serving.

If you have listened closely this week, perhaps you can already define "severely handicapped persons." A severe handicap means a disability that requires multiple services over an extended period of time. The disability results from amputation, blindness, carcinoma, cerebral palsy, cystic fibrosis, deafness, heart disease, hemiplegia, mental retardation, mental illness, multiple sclerosis, muscular dystrophy, neurological disorders including stroke and epilepsy, paraplegia, quadriplegia, and other spinal cord problems, renal failure, respiratory or pulmonary dysfunction, and any other disabilities specified by the Secretary of HEW in the regulations he shall prescribe. Well, what's left out? The term "severely impaired" includes each one of these diseases or impaired categories. Now, if you really look at the list, you may say, "Bill, what isn't severe anymore?"

I must relate another story to clarify the working counselor's position. In North Georgia, besides the processing of corn into a liquid state there is another great vocational endeavor, the raising of chickens. A friend of mine came to the foot of the hills one day and told his son and another boy, "I want you to go out and get a good, long, stout stick. I want one of you to sit on the front of this truckload of chickens, and I want one of you to sit on the back. When I start up the hill and blow the horn twice, want both of you to flail those cages just as hard as you can." The man's son said, "Well, Daddy, what in the world do you want us to do that for?" He said, "Well, son, this is a one-ton truck. We're going to haul two tons of chickens across that mountain. When I start up the mountain and blow the horn, I want you to flail those cages so hard that half of those chickens will be flying and the other half will not be flying. We have a one-ton truck, so if one ton of those chickens is flying and the other ton's in the cages, we'll make it over the hill." Now, many of you, as counselors, feel like you are carrying five tons in a one-ton truck. However, I will say to you that from the image you have gained among your peers, as well as within the region, the administration must feel you are capable of hauling five tons with a one-ton workload. I do not doubt that we as counselors will meet this role in Tennessee and in any other state. The problem is that if you just have the time, the clients will be served.

Now, let's get down to what each one of you is faced with every day. This is your problem, and I think many of you have heard why you are doing this and why you are going to continue to do it. Many of you have had the process explained to you, but let's look at what you are faced with as counselor. I want to approach the process in its three stages: referral, provision of services, and closure. In regard to referral, what type of client do you usually receive? I know that there are many of you in this audience who have used the Georgia Warm Springs Hospital, which is now a part of Georgia Vocational Rehabilitation. Although the Georgia Rehabilitation Center has been operated for years by Vocational Rehabilitation ,the hospital had not. Since July 7, 1974, the Georgia Warm Springs Hospital, a physical restoration institution serving the spinal cord injured, the amputee, the arthritic, and the epileptic, has been under our State Vocational Rehabilitation Operation. Let me tell you what I have encountered in the eleven years at the hospital—eleven years that are included in the fifteen years that I have been in rehabilitation. I spent five years as a counselor. I remember when I first started with a caseload. You know how it is when you are new and go into a new territory. Everybody from every other agency, including physicians, has been saving his favorite cases. Every counselor preceding you has tried to take them on the caseload. Now, this client would usually have been someone in the forty to fifty age range; he had usually worked hard as a laborer all of his life. All of a sudden he was rendered severely impaired. Many of you know the process you would go through, a process that includes reports from the doctor, health nurse, welfare officer, and so forth. In all honesty ,these clients are not the ones you are going to rehabilitate in six months, eighteen months, or possibly three years. When you go into the territory, someone from the hospital calls you and says, "You're just the individual I've been looking for. You rehabilitation counselors are the saviors of the world." While he's patting you on the back, you can feel the other thing gently sliding in at the same time. When he gets through with the "buttering up" you think, "Oh, yes I am marvelous, and I am good, and I think I will have some money to work with." Then he says, "By the way, I have a paraplegic over here, and I'd like you to take him on your caseload." Yo do take him on the caseload and you know what you are faced with. We have found that age, education, and work history background have been some of the problems of the severely impaired. A paraplegic is really not a rehabilitation problem. Many of you know you could place him in training if his age and education were such that he could pass the test necessary to get him into the various training programs. We have been trying to obtain monies from other agencies. In Georgia, we have attempted to work through the SSI and the SSDI. In Tennessee, I understand, this is either started or will be stated soon, primarily through the involvement of Workman's Compensation.

There are also personal and social situations. I have alluded very briefly to the family problem. You know that your severely impaired client is not the only one with whom you counsel. You also counsel the family members. You counsel the employer. You counsel with everyone associated with the client more than you counsel with the client himself. There are a multiplicity of problems that result from a severe impairment. Severe impairments have produced home breakups and untold emotional damage to many families. For example, when you make a home visit, what is the reaction of the family members? Can any of you think of a particular situation with which you have been faced? With whom did you end up talking? I guarantee you it wasn't that poor client. This individual is wondering if it's even worth living because he has looked at what he once had and what he does not have now.

For instance, I was counseling at the hospital one day. This man had been a drag line operator. He hit a power line running along an open ditch that he was dragging. When his bucket came into contact with the electrical line, this man literally lost both legs above the knees and both arms above the elbow from the electric shock. He spent about eight months in a general hospital lying in bed. In addition to losing all four extremities, he had developed pressure sores, or decubitus ulcers, on the bony prominences of his hips. This man was ridden with infection. I went over as the "friendly rehabilitation counselor." He was lying in bad and I said, "Good morning, I'm Bill Tomlin." He said, "So what?" I said "Do you know who I am?" and he said, "No, and I don't give a damn." I was saying to myself that this client wasn't very cooperative. He asked me what I wanted and said "Are you a preacher?" I said, "No, I'm not a preacher." He said, "Are you a doctor?" and I said, "No, I'm not a doctor either." Then, he said, "Well, what do you do?" I tried to think fast about what a rehabilitation counselor does and I said, "I'm here to help you get back to work." He said, "Young man, you should be in Central State Hospital." Central State Hospital is our large mental institution. Then he said, "How could some fool come in here? Here I am with no legs, no arms, eaten up with bed sores, and you're talking about work?" I said "Yes sir." Then he said, "You're crazy, sir. You need electroshock bad."

That is not the rare case. Many of you are faced with the same kind of client every day. In all this depression, he and I finally found a base. The base was that he had been a productive individual, and he had a very loving wife and three children. He was the one who was trying to drop them. Now believe it or not, this is where you get into counseling. The preacher, the pastor in your church, tells you he doesn't want to get into it. The doctor very warily tells you it is not his problem. It boils down to whose problem it is. It's the rehabilitation counselor's problem, and we accept it. That's something I am proud to say. I don't know a rehabilitation counselor who will run from any case. We get a lot of services passed over to us, but if we don't that person would possibly never get any service. When you're talking with an individual who has given up, you're going to spend a lot of time trying to convince him that it's worth living. When you reach this point, you can start counseling about work. This particular individual had electronics ability. We fitted him with upper extremity prostheses that had multiple types of attachments. Now he is working at an electronics assembly plant doing electronic sub-assembly. We also fitted him with two above-knee prostheses. The last time I heard the man was still working.

Many of you can remember the day that you approached some severely impaired person. You can recall where the process starts, and all you have to go through with a client to get him to the point where he will enter into a full time rehabilitation program. You must also take into consideration the fact that funds from insurance, workmen's compensation, SSI, SSDI, joint VRPA grants, private groups ,or even civic groups may not be available. Unless things are different here than in our state, you're not running over with case money. You are probably spending half of your yearly allotment right now, even though the fiscal year has barely started.

I think that at this time I will cut short my presentation to give time to Dr. William Graves. I know some material he has added that I think will go in line with what I have been saying. I want to close with reference to one thing. After you have provided physical restoration, evaluation, and training, your real job is going to be continued counseling in the home about job placement. You provide excellent rehabilitation and physical restoration services and training for job preparation. However, if you don't have a home environment where the individual has a family that is willing to get up at 5:30 every morning, bathe, dress, feed, and transport the person to the job—or if you don't set up some medical follow-up for the severely impaired, even after closure—I can assure you that you are going to have him right back in your caseload. These people will need more of your help at this time than they need in the hospital or in rehabilitation centers. I will say to you, "Be aware." The ones of you who have really gone through this process with severely impaired people now realize that your real counseling job takes place after the client gets home. You start the placement and the continued care at home.

I would close with just one more notation. I served three rural counties for five years. I was extremely interested in the Heart Association, and Dr. W. B. Fackler, a cardiologist in my territory, sponsored my membership in the American and Georgia Heart Association Rehabilitation Council. One day Dr. Fackler called me at the employment office and said, "Bill, I want you to come over and see this man." I said, "Well, Dr. Fackler, I'd be glad to. What's the trouble?" He said, "The man is dying," and I said, "Well, isn't it a little late for a referal to a rehabilitation counselor?" He said, "Bill, what I want you to do is counsel with this client. We have had no success. Nobody can communicate with this man. We just want you to talk to him." "Oh," I said, "now you are in my field; if there's one thing I can do, I can talk." So I went to the hospital. Dr. Fackler and the nurses were there with this cardiac case. There were tubes down his nose, and tubes in his throat; machines were pumping; and the man was just lying there. I said, "Well, Dr. Fackler, let me try." He said, "If you can just get some spark of life out of him . . ." I said, "Okay, I'll give it a try." So I walked over to the bed, and I started talking to this man. All of a sudden there was a facial expression. I thought "Now I have established rapport. I have a real communication link with this man. The doctors and all the other people couldn't even communicate with this person." Then the man raised his arms. The doctors said, "My gosh, Bill, you even have him moving." Then I was going. I turned on. The patient pointed to the desk where there was a pencil and pad. They handed it to him, and he wrote something. Just as he finished the last line, he dropped, and he died. Well, I was about one of the most despondent counselors you have ever seen in your life. As I was standing there near the bed, I looked at the paper. This man had written: "You damn fool; you're standing on my oxygen line." The moral of this story is: as counselors serving impaired people—although you feel like you are working with more than you can do—please don't stand on a severely impaired person's oxygen line. Give him the benefit of your very excellent rehabilitation counseling services. Thank you.

William H. Graves

Strategies for Counseling
the Severely Disabled

Counseling theories such as client-centered and Gestalt are developed on populations decidedly different from groups served by rehabilitation counselors. Such theories are felt to be inappropriate for use by those counselors working with the severely disabled, especially those from poor or lower-class backgrounds. Dr. Graves describes this rehabilitation client and such a client's reasons for seeking counseling. A model for prescriptive counseling is explained.

Multiple sclerosis, rheumatoid arthritis, multiple amputations, strokes, hemiplegia, paraplegia, quadriplegia, blindness, deafness, cerebral palsy, epilepsy—all are severe disabilities. All interrupt the normal developmental process. Some assault the man in the street, some the developing fetus, others the marvelous young athlete racing toward victory. Deafness, for example, interferes with communication and, as a consequence, has profound effects on academic achievement. In 1973, the average academic achievement level for a graduate of the Mississippi School of the Deaf was less than the fifth grade. Amputations affect mobility and appearance and apparently can interfere with typical social behaviors. Rusk and Taylor report that 50 per cent of the college students surveyed would not date a person who had an amputated leg, and 65 per cent would not marry an amputee.[1] Severe disability also affects emotional well-being. Kir-Stimon writes that "There is, among these people, a deep sense of being forlorn, alienated from the rest of the world."[2]

Severe disability can and does have profound effects on the life of any individual. But severe disability has an even more serious and profound effect on the individual who is from the lower or working class or from an impoverished background. Let me continue Kir-Stimon's paragraph to illustrate this point:

... There is, among these people, a deep sense of being forlorn, alienated from the rest of the world; the individual is hemmed in physically, usually more than he has ever been in his entire life, a hemming in from which he

225

knows he canot be extricated ... and for the most part, he can no longer express himself in any significant physical movement ....[3]

It is this lack of significant movement, this freezing of body language, this sudden muting of the stamping foot that increasingly burdens the severely disabled who also happen to be poor. The poor rely heavily on a restrictive code of language which depends often on non-verbal codes to communicate personal identity statements.[4] They cannot use verbiage to communicate with the middle-class counselor. Hence, the rehabilitation counseling process will be frustrated because the counselor and client are not communicating. It is like a Kafka short story: two people playing checkers, but playing by different rules; no one wins, and no one loses; only craziness. Carkhuff and Berenson write that "If counselors and psychotherapists functioned in real life the way most of them do in the therapeutic hour they would be patients."[5] We rehabilitation counselors in Tennessee and the Southeast need to consider the effects of poverty and the lower-class culture on the severely disabled and their implications for providing rehabilitation services to our clients, most of whom are poor or from a lower-class background. Seldom are SSI referrals not poor or not from a lower-class background, and the majority can be classified as severely disabled. The severely disabled cannot be considered independently of their culture.

Most counseling theories have been developed on populations decidedly different from the clients that you rehabilitation counselors see in your offices, in their homes, at the post office, welfare office, or where have you. Psychoanalysis was developed on upper-middle-class Jewish women in central Europe. I haven't seen one yet in a rehabilitation counselor's office! Client-centered counseling is not appropriate for most clients seen by the vocational rehabilitation counselor. It is not appropriate because the skills required of the client to successfully benefit from client-centered counseling are not possessed by most vocational rehabilitation clients. Let me give you an example of what happened to me when I used client-centered counseling inappropriately.

When I received my master's degree in rehabilitation counseling in 1965, classic client-centered counseling was the major approach emphasized by counselor education programs. Like all good, fresh master's graduates, I took what I learned as appropriate counseling behavior for all clients into my field office. So one day, a lady came in to see me in a desperate situation. She was a dental technician. She was having problems standing. Her biggest problem in standing was that one leg was slightly shorter than the other and her standing caused pain in the hip. The surgeon suggested surgery. The difference in the heights of the legs could be resolved, and she would be able to stand without pain. It sounded like a very simple physical restoration case. Well, I approached it in a very client-centered fashion. I let her make the decision to go into surgery, and this sounded fine. She'd get along fine. The doctor promised me she'd be able to go back to work in six weeks. Fine. Well, it didn't work out that way. Hip surgeries seldom do. She wasn't able to go back to work in six weeks. One of the things I neglected to investigate was her family problems. She was separated. She was living with her kids in public housing. The kids ranged from about five to about fifteen years of age. The father was in another city, and when she went into the hospital she had no source of income. Well, first of all I was too stupid, and I don't know any other word to use, to see if we could provide some income for the woman during the period of hospitalization and recuperation. In the state in which I was working only welfare could provide maintenance and support during this period. Rehabilitation monies in that state were not available to provide maintenance or support during periods of hospitalization. Welfare would not provide her any money, primarily because she was eligible for child support from her husband, except that the husband didn't want to pay child support. The answer, of course, was for her to sue for child support. She wanted to do that, but her kids said, "No, you ain't gonna put my Daddy in jail." Well, somehow, the kids survived and they made it through the hospitalization. One day she came into my office. She was extremely agitated, crying, and angry; I've never seen a person angrier. I was listening to her talk and I started saying in my best reflective style, "Yes, ma'am, I understand. You're really angry, aren't you?" She said, "Hell, yes, I'm angry. Stop playing this silly damn game of saying everything I say over again and do something!" I realized that I wasn't communicating with this woman; I was being a professional college counselor. I wasn't serving this woman. Then I finally got off my rear end and decided to provide some services to this woman instead of being a reflective client-centered counselor. We got her into a rehabilitation facility that day, which I should have done anyway, provided some maintenance, and she began work conditioning. About six months later, she was able to return to her job. A simple case, I admit, but I tried to use some counseling techniques that were inappropriate, and disaster resulted.

Many counseling models that you've been taught in graduate school are not appropriate for our clients. Most counseling models have been developed on this kind of people: YAVIS. YAVIS people are Young, Attractive, Verbal, Intelligent, and Successful.[6] If they have those five characteristics, they aren't rehab clients. When theories are developed on one population, they typically are effective for that population. Client-centered counseling does work for college students; it's excellent. Psychoanalysis does work for upper middle-class people. Gestalt counseling, which is one of the latest models, does work for alienated, liberal, frustrated people of the 1970's, but it is not going to work for rehab clients who don't share the characteristics of the population on which the techniques were developed.

Rehabilitation counselors, by and large, work with clients who are non-YAVIS: working or poor, middle aged or elderly, physically ordinary or unattractive, verbally reticent, intellectually unexceptional or dull, and vocationally unsuccessful or marginal. Our clients behave differently from the YAVIS clients. They seek counseling because of specific, immediate, and concrete problems related to their environment which they are unable to resolve. They come to you because they want something now. It's very specific: "I want a job. I can't find a job. Nobody will hire me because. . . ." Usually they can't resolve this problem themselves so they come to you for some help. Usually they come to you because someone in their environment who is important to them, such as a preacher, a doctor, a nurse, or a welfare officer, tells them that they need counseling and this man at the rehab agency can help them. When they come to you, they are seeking immediate relief from the stress they are experiencing. They want relief now, not next week or next year. They state their problems, then assume a passive role: "Mr. Graves, I can't find a job. Nobody will hire me. Will you get me one?" And that's the end of it. They want a job. They anticipate that the counselor will offer advice and guide them to a solution of their problems. They seek help in a different kind of way than the way most of the counseling theories and models offer help. The typical verbally-oriented counseling theories state that the client should be responsible for being active in the counseling relationship. Non-YAVIS clients aren't like that. They expect that you will give them advice and guide them to solve their problems.

Rehabilitation counseling for the non-YAVIS, severely disabled client is a teaching process. It's an educational process. Most importantly, I believe that you should not approach these clients from a disease point of view. I'm saying they're not sick. I'm saying that they lack some skills that you can teach them so that they can cope more effectively. Rehabilitation counseling can be a teaching process based on individualized instruction. The vocational rehabilitation model is excellent in helping you do your job of teaching the client certain coping skills. It provides a process that allows the rehabilitation counselor to *prescribe* the services needed by this severely handicapped person to achieve his vocational rehabilitation goal.

Rehabilitation counseling is basically prescriptive counseling. The client is evaluated to identify his problems and alternative solutions to the problems. The counselor, as he works with the client, is able to prescribe the best solutions to the problems. This model allows for continual evaluation, feedback, maximum client involvement, and community services. It provides a rehabilitation facility where counselors, evaluators, personal adjustment counselors, supervisors, and technicians can develop specific individual prescriptions to allow non-YAVIS severely disabled clients to develop success skills that will in turn allow them to achieve vocational adjustment.

Notes

1. H. A. Rusk and E. J. Taylor, *New Hope for the Handicapped* (New York: Harper & Row, 1946).

2. William Kir-Stimon, "Conseling with the Severely Handicapped—Encounter and Commitments," *Psychotherapy: Theory, Research and Practice*, Vol. 7 (1970).

3. *Ibid.*

4. B. Bernstein, *Social Class and Linguistic Development: A Theory of Social Learning* (New York: Free Press, 1961).

5. R. R. Carkhuff and B. G. Berenson, *Beyond Counseling and Therapy* (New York: Holt, Rinehart & Winston, 1967).

6. A. P. Goldstein, *Structured Learning Therapy: Toward a Psychotherapy for the Poor* (New York: Academic Press, 1973).

7. *Ibid.*

William M. Jenkins, Robert M. Anderson
and Wilson L. Dietrich

Conclusions and Implications

A four-day conference which focused on services for severely disabled clients was conducted August 26-29, 1974, at the Holiday Inn Rivermont, Memphis, Tennessee. The purpose of the conference was to bring together rehabilitation personnel for interpretation of the Rehabilitation Act of 1973 and to provide a training program to increase and improve services for the more severely handicapped clients.

The agenda for the conference included a variety of lectures, panel discussions, and other activities. Each participant received travel reimbursement including per diem, hotel expense, and mileage reimbursement.

Following the conference an evaluation form was completed by each participant (see Appendix C). The following questions and responses exemplify the types of items utilized in the evaluation form and the comments made by the conference participants. The questions, which were answered by "yes" or "no" responses, are shown in Table I. A wide majority of the participants responded positively.

Participants were asked to rate the program and the instructors on a continuum ranging from "poor" to "excellent." The responses are shown in Table II. Again, the responses are quite positive.

The respondents were asked to indicate the topics they felt would benefit them most. As might have been predicted, the summarization and interpretation of the Rehabilitation Act of 1973 was considered to be the most beneficial to most of the participants. While all of the topics were considered to be relevant to the needs of the participants, the four topics which were most frequently cited were:

1. Rehabilitation Act of 1973
2. Medical and Psycho-Social Problems of the Spinal-Cord Injured Client

TABLE I
Attitudes Toward Program Planning

Questions	Yes	No
Was the course basically what you expected?	149	22
Was appropriate time devoted to each topic?	137	22
Were you and other participants allowed adequate opportunity to participate and ask questions?	153	11
Was advance publicity adequate?	132	25
Were registration procedures adequate?	157	3
Were facilities adequate?	142	18

TABLE II
Program and Instructors Ratings

Questions	Excellent	Good	Fair	Poor
Would you rate the program as	62	74	26	6
Would you rate the instructor(s) as	61	85	20	3

3. Counselor Certification
4. Counseling Strategies with the Severely Disabled

The participants were given an opportunity to make general comments about the conference. Space does not permit a complete listing of all comments and suggestions. The following responses are representative:

"Program was relevant, useful and timely. It was well-organized and professionally administered."

"An excellent conference. Memphis State University did a very good job in putting it together."

"A very good conference—one of the best I have attended since being with VR."

"Well organized—instructors and speakers were good."

"A good conference—considering the number of people at the meeting. I would like to have seen more small group sessions."

"Program was much better than others I have attended. The emphasis on severely handicapped was much needed and should show a beneficial effect in the attitudes and work of the counselors."

"I feel that this was the best inservice training I have attended. I do hope that we have opportunities like the conference in Memphis again. It was extremely worthwhile. Of course, I would have liked some emphasis to have been given to deafness."

"The program was well organized. Speakers were people who could speak with authority in their areas of expertise. Conference area was easy to get to. The only thing I missed was more opportunity to participate in small groups for professional discussion."

"This was an excellent meeting. It was well organized and very helpful."

"Program Committee should be congratulated for pulling together such a reality based, mind stretching faculty. The best training I've attended. Learned a lot and enjoyed it."

"Above average—felt like there should have been some time devoted to the Mental Health program and to mental health problems since one in ten is affected."

"This was one of the better inservice training programs that I have attended."

"This was without a doubt one of the best inservice training programs I have attended."

"I have heard only good comments about the sessions from our disability examiners who attended."

"Very relevant meeting—severely disabled is our mandate."

In summary, there was a strong consensus that the inservice training program had been productive and that similar workshops should be conducted on a regular basis in the future.

Appendix A

Program Participants

Armstrong, Cheryl, President of Tennessee Vocational Evaluation and Work Adjustment Association, Memphis Goodwill, Memphis, Tennessee

Batchelor, Roy, Division of Special Assignments, Department of Education, Nashville, Tennessee

Baxter, Russell, Commissioner of Rehabilitation Services, Department of Social and Rehabilitation Services, Little Rock, Arkansas

Brown, Herbert L., Director of Disability Determinations, Disability Determinations Section, Division of Vocational Rehabilitation, Nashville, Tennessee

Bynum, Richard F., Assistant Professor, Disability Examiner Education, University of Tennessee, Knoxville, Tennessee

Carmichael, D. Benjamin E., Commissioner of Education, Department of Education, Nashville, Tennessee

Chadwick, Judge Richard C., Administrative Law Judge, Bureau of Hearings & Appeals, Department of Health, Education, and Welfare, Memphis, Tennessee

Childs, Richard N., Supervisor of Work-Study Programs, Division of Vocational Rehabilitation, Nashville, Tennessee

Couch, Dr. Robert, Coordinator of Rehabilitation and Special Edution Programs, Auburn University, Auburn, Alabama

Countryman, Gwen, National President, NARS, Little Rock, Arkansas

Davis, Lewis, Associate Regional Representative for Rehabilitation Services, Atlanta, Georgia

Dietrich, Dr. Wilson, Chairman, Department of Special Education and Rehabilitation, Memphis State University, Memphis, Tennessee

Duncan, Jack, Counsel, Select Sub-Committee on Education, U.S. House of Representatives, Washington, D.C.

Fanning, Milton H., Director of Management Services, Division of Vocational Rehabilitation, Nashville, Tennessee

Gaines, Tom, National President of VEWAA, Division of Vocational Rehabilitation, Fayetteville, N.C.

Graves, Dr. Bill, Coordinator of Rehabilitation Counselor Education, Mississippi State University, Starkville, Mississippi

Griffin, Clint, Counselor, Division of Vocational Rehabilitation, Nashville, Tennessee

Haddle, Dr. Harold W., Jr., Psychologist, Georgia Mental Health Institute, Atlanta, Georgia

Hansen, Dr. Carl, Coordinator of Rehabilitation Counselor Education, University of Texas, Austin, Texas

Huerka, Pearl, Southeast Region President, NARS, Tampa, Florida

Jenkins, Dr. William M., Coordinator of Rehabilitation Counselor Education, Memphis State University, Memphis, Tennessee

Jones, Dr. Billy M., President of Memphis State University, Memphis, Tennessee

Lee, Frank E., Administrative Assistant, Division of Vocational Rehabilitation, Nashville, Tennessee

McLelland, Shelton W., Retired Association Regional Commissioner for Rehabilitation Services, Atlanta, Georgia

Mills, Craig, Director of Florida Division of Vocational Rehabilitation, Tallahassee, Florida

Mirring, Paul, Field Coordinator of NARC On-the-Job Training Project, Atlanta, Georgia

Moore, Carroll, Director of Disability Determinations Unit 2, Disability Determination Service, Division of Vocational Rehabilitation, Nashville, Tennessee

Morgan, Dr. Clayton, Coordinator, Rehabilitation Counselor Education, Oklahoma State University, Stillwater, Oklahoma

Owens, Joseph, Council of State Administrators of Vocational Rehabilitation, Washington, D.C.

Reece, O. E. Assistant Commissioner of the Division of Vocational Rehabilitation, Nashville, Tennessee

Saunders, Dr. Robert, Dean of the College of Education, Memphis State University, Memphis, Tennessee

Sax, Dr. Arnold B., Director, Materials Development Center, University of Wisconsin-Stout, Menomonie, Wisconsin

Smits, Dr. Stan, Coordinator, Rehabilitation Counselor Education Program, Georgia State University, Atlanta, Georgia

Steede, Kitty, State Chapter President, NARS, Nashville, Tennessee

Tomlin, William A., Southeast Regional President of NRCA, Warm Springs, Georgia

Tooms, Robert E., M.D., The Campbell Clinic, Inc., Memphis, Tennessee

Van Hooser, Jack, Director of Manpower and Planning, Division of Vocational Rehabilitation, Nashville, Tennessee

Walker, Betty Ann, National President-Elect of NARS

Walker, Robyn S., Supervisor of Case Services, Division of Vocational Rehabilitation, Knoxville, Tennessee

Wiggins, Greer, Manager of Vocational Training Center, Murfreesboro, Tennessee

Williams, Martha Gene, President-Elect, VSRA, Chattanooga, Tennessee

Williams, William M., Director, Division of Vocational Rehabilitation, Nashville, Tennessee

Wright, Bill, Wage Analyst, U.S. Department of Labor, Nashville, Tennessee

APPENDIX B

MATERIALS ACCOMPANYING BEHAVIOR CHANGE THROUGH SELF-CONTROL

ADAPTIVE SOCIETY   MALADAPTIVE ANXIETY

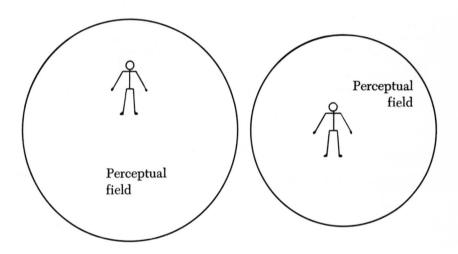

Minimum of anxiety, openness to environment, perceptual field open, high level of awareness, in touch with reality.

Overwhelming anxiety, closed to environment, perceptual field blocked, low level of awareness, distortion of reality.

FIGURE 1

CHART I
Anxiety Indicator Chart

	Level	Mental State	Physical State
Beta	100	wide awake	uptight
	90	high sensory awareness	moist, clammy hands
	80	aware and active	hyperactivity
	70	comfortable and alert	restful state
	60	thought patterns normal	restful physically
	50	thoughts less active	more composure
Alpha	40	increased susceptibility	passively aware
	30	total sensory withdrawal	deep relaxation
Theta	20	drowsy	no awareness
	10	unconscious	unconscious
Delta	5	deep sleep	deep sleep
	0		

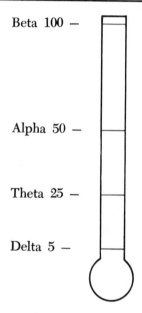

Beta 100 —

Alpha 50 —

Theta 25 —

Delta 5 —

(Thermometer Model)

RELAXATION EXERCISES

Get really comfortable. Settle back in your chair, and relax as much as possible. Close your eyes. Take a few deep breaths, and begin to feel yourself let go. With your head resting on the back of your chair and your arms resting on the arms of the chair let the support of your body be given by the chair. Do not let your body muscles support your body. Now while you relax the rest of your body, clinch your right fist. Clinch it tighter and tighter. Notice the tension. Keep it clinched. (5 seconds) In your fist, hand, and forearm notice the tension. Notice the difference in the tension in your right hand, fist, and forearm, in contrast to the relaxation in the rest of your body. Now relax. Allow your right hand to become loose; allow it to completely relax. Let it fall down beside your body. Notice especially the contrast in feeling in moving from the tension to relaxation. Learn to appreciate the difference. Now let your whole body become more and more relaxed. Just enjoy the relaxation.

Left fist. Now, repeat the tension with your left fist. Squeeze it tightly. Squeeze it tighter and tighter. Feel the tension in your fist, hand, and forearm. Now while you relax the rest of your body notice the difference between the tension and the relaxation. Clinch your fist tighter and tighter. Notice the tension in your left hand, fist, and forearm in contrast to the relaxation in the rest of your body. Now relax. Allow your left hand to become loose—allow it to completely relax. Let it fall down beside your body. Notice especially the contrast now that you are feeling moving from the tension to relaxation. Appreciate the difference. Now let your whole body become more and more relaxed. Just enjoy the relaxation.

Continue relaxing once more. Notice the nice, warm feeling that you experience as you relax. Study the differences now between the feelings of relaxation and the tension you just experienced.

Both fists. Now, clinch both fists. While the rest of your body relaxes clinch both fists. Notice the tension in your forearms, fists, and wrists. (5 seconds)

Now, relax your fists. Let your fingers fall loose. Notice how different it is to relax in contrast to the tension. Just sit back, and allow your entire body to relax. Your forearms, fists, and wrists are beginning to feel heavier as the relaxation spreads throughout them. (5 seconds)

Biceps. O.K., fine. Now let's concentrate on the biceps. Bend your elbows, and tense the bicep muscles in both arms. Feel the tension in your biceps. Contrast it to the relaxation in the rest of your body. (5 seconds) Now, relax your arms. Allow the relaxation to spread deeper and deeper. Attend to the heavy, warm feelings associated with the relaxation as they spread all the way to the tips of your fingers. Continue to relax, deeper and deeper.

Triceps. Now, straighten out your arms. Feel the tension in your triceps. (5 seconds) Now, relax again. Learn to enjoy the warm feelings of relaxation. Let the relaxation develop on its own. Let yourself relax more freely and deeply, and let the relaxation spread up your arms until they feel heavier and heavier—enjoyably heavier. Relax more and more; try to go deeper and deeper, further and further—to a deeper level of relaxation.

Face, neck, shoulders. Now we will concentrate on your face, neck, and shoulders. Let's concentrate first on the muscles in your forehead. Wrinkle up your forehead, frown. Raise your eyebrows— more and more—while the rest of your body relaxes. Make it tighter and tighter. (5 seconds) Now relax. Let the muscles smooth out and become smoother and smoother.

O.K. Let's work on your eyes. Close them tightly. Make them tighter and tighter. Feel the tension. (5 seconds) Pay attention to the difference between the tension in your eyes and the relaxation in the rest of your body. Now relax. Keep your eyes closed and notice the soothing, calm feeling in your eyes.

Mouth. Now let's work on the area around your mouth. Bite your teeth together. (5 seconds) Feel the tension in your jaws. Feel your throat muscles get tight. Feel the tension become greater as you bite your teeth together. Now relax. Let your jaw, eyes, and forehead relax.

Lips. Draw the corners of your moth back—try to grin from ear to ear. (5 seconds) Now relax. Let your jaw hang loose. Again appreciate the feeling of relaxation. Notice the difference between the tension and relaxation. Notice how much more regular your breathing is becoming, as you become more deeply relaxed.

Tongue. Now, press hard against the roof of your mouth with your tongue. Study the tension there. Notice how the tension mounts as you press it against the roof of your mouth. (5 seconds) Now relax.

Let your tongue fall loose. Feel the relaxation come over you, come over your whole body as you allow yourself to become more deeply relaxed. Just enjoy it . . . enjoy the wonderful relaxation feelings all over your body. (5 seconds)

Neck. Now, press your head back as far as it will go. Hold it there. Now press your chin forward and down against your chest. Hold this. (5 seconds) Now move your head to its normal position. Let your neck be loose. Feel the relief you experience by letting your neck become loose. Continue to enjoy the beautiful relaxation. (5 seconds)

Shoulders. Good, now let's concentrate on your shoulder muscles. Shrug your shoulders, and try to touch your ears. (5 seconds) Push hard. Notice the tension. (5 seconds) Now relax. Let your shoulders slump, and attend to the nice, warm, tingling feelings as they spread throughout your shoulders. Let these feelings spread through to your arms, then all the way down to the tips of your fingers. Let it also spread into your face, throat, and jaws. Let the relaxation spread all over . . . . Let it grow deeper and deeper. Become aware of the pleasant, heavy feelings all over your body as you relax.

Chest, stomach, lower back.

Chest. Take a deep breath. Fill your lungs with air. Notice the tension in your chest. Now exhale—let it out—breathe normally now. Notice how you breathe. Let your chest fall loose as you feel the relaxation spread throughout your chest and the rest of your body. Just enjoy this relaxation. Take another deep breath. Hold it as you breathe it in. Now, let it out. Enjoy it. Notice the difference in the relief of exhaling, breathing rhythmically as you give over to the relaxation more and more. Let yourself go . . . feel the relaxation in your neck, shoulders, and chest.

Stomach. Now pay attention to your stomach. Tighten your abdomen muscles. Make your abdomen hard. Press it tighter and tighter. Pay attention to the tension. Now relax. Just let your stomach muscles go. Breathe regularly. As you breathe out and in, your stomach relaxes more and more. Now, suck it in so you try to touch your backbone with it. (5 seconds) Now relax. Notice the rhythmic breathing now. Try to let go more and more. Let your body sink more and more into the chair by letting it relax further and further.

Lower back. Pay attention now to your lower back. Arch your

back more and more. Feel the tension in this area. Contrast it to the relaxation in the rest of your body. (5 seconds) Now relax. Feel the tingling relaxation feelings in many parts of your body as you:

Relax your stomach, relax your lower back, your chest, your shoulders, your neck, your face, your arms, and your hands.

Let the relaxation continue to proceed on it own—deeper and deeper. Enjoy the feelings as these parts of your body relax further and further.

Hips, thighs, calves.

Hips, Shift your attention now to your hip muscles. Tense your buttocks muscles. Do this by pressing your heels down to the floor. (5 seconds) Now relax. Let the relaxation proceed on its own. Enjoy the nice relaxing feelings as you relax deeper and deeper.

Thighs. Now, lift and stretch your right leg out. Tense the muscles in your right thigh. Push out as hard as you can. Now let your right leg fall slowly into place. Attend to the relief and comfort you experience as your leg relaxes—as your entire body relaxes.

Now lift your left leg. Stretch it out. Tense the thigh muscles. Feel the tension mount. Now, allow your left leg to drop slowing into place. Attend to the relief and comfort your experience as your leg relaxes.

Feel now the pleasantness of the relaxation as it spreads throughout your body. Let it proceed as you become more and more relaxed. Now lift and stretch both legs. Straight out. Tense the thigh muscles again. (5 seconds) Now let both legs relax.

Calves. Now, let's pay attention to your calf muscles. Push toes on both legs down—as far as you can. (5 seconds) Relax. Now press down again, tensing the calf muscles. (5 seconds) Now up again. Relax.

Now, press your toes upward with your heels on the floor. Point them toward your face—flex the calf muscles. (5 seconds) Relax again. Experience the nice warm feelings of relaxation. Press your toes upward again, toward your face with your heels on the floor. Notice the tension. Now, relax them, and allow the relaxation to spread all over your legs and the rest of your body.

I will indicate the different parts of your body to help you relax better. This time don't tense these parts but just relax them further and further. Try to get that extra bit of relaxation in each muscle group as I mention it:

Feet relax (5 seconds)
Ankles relax (5 seconds)
Calves relax (5 seconds)
Thighs relax (5 seconds)
Buttocks relax (5 seconds)
Hips relax (5 seconds)

Feel the pleasantness of the relaxation in the lower parts of your body as you relax further and further. Now relax these parts of your body:

Lower back relax (5 seconds)
Stomach relax (5 seconds)
Chest relax (5 seconds)
Shoulders relax (5 seconds)
Mouth relax (5 seconds)
Eyes relax (5 seconds)
Forehead relax (5 seconds)
Arms relax (5 seconds)
Hands relax (5 seconds)

All the way to the tips of your fingers, relax. Let the relaxation take over freely. Let all your muscles relax. From the top of your head to the tips of your toes, relax. Carry on the relaxation now—just enjoy relaxing. (2 minutes)

Now, please, as I count from 4 to 1, stretch and yawn and open your eyes. Four, three, two, one.